Sirt Food
Diet Cookbook

~400~

Quick & Easy Sirt Recipes To Burn Fat by Activating Your "Skinny Gene"

Serena Baxter

TABLE OF CONTENTS

INTRODUCTION		6
APPETIZER AND SNACK RECIPES		7
1.	Fruit Salad	7
2.	Golden Turmeric Latte	7
3.	The Sirt Juice	7
4.	Kale Pesto Hummus	7
5.	Parsley Hummus	8
6.	Edamame Hummus	8
7.	Edamame Guacamole	8
8.	Eggplant Fries with Fresh Aioli	9
9.	Eggplant Caponata	9
10.	Buckwheat Crackers	9
11.	Matcha Protein Bites	10
12.	Chocolate-Covered Strawberry Trail Mix	10
13.	Moroccan Spiced Eggs	10
14.	Exquisite Turmeric Pancakes with Lemon Yogurt Sauce	11
15.	Sirt Chili Con Carne	12
16.	Med-Style Olives	12
17.	Crispy Chickpeas	12
18.	Honey Chili Nuts	12
19.	Cauliflower Nachos	13
20.	Cheesy Cauliflower Bars	13
21.	Walnut and Date Bites	13
22.	Sirt Energy Balls	13
23.	Celery and Raisins Snack Salad	14
24.	Yogurt & Fruit Jam Parfait	14
25.	Lemon Ricotta Cookies	14
26.	Matcha Mochi	14
27.	Blueberry Muffins	15
28.	Brownie Bites	15
29.	Mascarpone Cheesecake	15
30.	Chocolate Berry Blend	16
31.	Monkey Trail Mix	16
32.	Granola with Quinoa	16
33.	Med-Styled Olives	16
34.	Roasted Chickpeas	17
35.	Baked Root Veg Crisps	17
36.	Bubble and Squeak	17
37.	Thai Cucumber Salad	18
38.	Mushroom Risotto	18
39.	Cauliflower-Olive Salad	18
40.	Zucchini-Crusted Pizza	19
41.	Broccoli Salad	19
42.	Not-Quite-Middle-Eastern Salad	19
43.	Apple Cinnamon Oats Bowl	19
44.	Paleo Power Bread	20
45.	Buckwheat Protein Bread	20
BREAKFAST RECIPES		21
46.	Strawberry Muesli	21
47.	Sirtfood Omelet	21
48.	Sirtfood Diet Smoothie	21
49.	Yogurt, Berries, Walnuts and Dark Chocolate	21
50.	Seasoned Scrambled Eggs	22
51.	Asian Shrimp Stir-Fry Along with Buckwheat Noodles	22
52.	Miso and Sesame Glazed Tofu with Ginger and Chili Stir	22
53.	Turkey Escalope with Sage, Parsley & Capers	23
54.	Buckwheat Pancakes, Mushrooms, Red Onions, and Kale Salad	23
55.	Naan Bread with Baked Tofu and Cauliflower	24
56.	Sautéed Potatoes in Chicken Broth	24
57.	Classic Waldorf Salad	25
58.	Whole Wheat Pita	25
59.	Scrambled Tofu with Mushrooms	25
60.	Pasta with Smoked Salmon and Arugula	26
61.	Tofu with Cauliflower	26
62.	Indulgent Yoghurt	26
63.	Frozen Gazpacho	26
64.	Tomato Frittata	27
65.	Chicken with Kale and Chili Salsa	27
66.	Buckwheat Tuna Casserole	27
67.	Tuscan Stewed Beans	28
68.	Buckwheat Tabbouleh with Strawberries	28
69.	Scramble Tofu and Mushroom	29
70.	Kale Scramble	29
71.	Pancakes with Blackcurrant Compote	29
72.	Cinnamon Buckwheat Porridge	29
73.	Mushroom Scramble Egg	30
74.	Sirtfood Eggs and Mushroom	30
75.	Matcha Green Juice	30
76.	Berry Pancakes	31
77.	Pumpkin Pancakes	31
78.	Simple Waffles	31
79.	Green Veggies Quiche	32
80.	Tofu & Kale Omelet	32
81.	Kale, Chickpeas & Olives Salad	32
82.	Steak Salad	33
83.	Chicken & Orange Salad	33
84.	Buckwheat Burgers	34
85.	Sautéed Mushrooms	34
86.	Kale with Cranberries & Pine Nuts	34
87.	Tofu with Kale	35
88.	Buckwheat Pancakes	35
89.	Blueberry Waffles	35
90.	Tofu & Arugula Scramble	35
MAIN DISH RECIPES		37
91.	Aromatic Chicken Breast, Kale, Red Onion, and Salsa	37
92.	Kale and Red Onion Dal with Buckwheat	37
93.	Chargrilled Beef and Herb Roasted Potatoes	37
94.	Crunchy Braised Leeks	38
95.	Sweet and Sour Pan with Cashew Nuts	38
96.	Eggplant and Spinach Casserole	39
97.	Vegetarian Paleo Ratatouille	39
98.	Vegetarian Curry from the Crock Pot	39
99.	Fried Cauliflower Rice	40
100.	Fried Chicken and Broccolini	40
101.	Turkey with Cauliflower Couscous	40
102.	Chicken Thighs with Creamy Tomato Spinach Sauce	41
103.	Sirt Chili with Meat	41

#	Recipe	Page
104.	Chickpea, Quinoa and Turmeric Curry	42
105.	Chargrilled Beef with a Red Wine	42
106.	Creamy Beef and Shells	43
107.	Rowdy Enchiladas	43
108.	Braised Pork Belly and Avocado Skewers	44
109.	Chicken Ayam	44
110.	Sri Lankan-Style Sweet Potato Curry	44
111.	Chicken Liver Along with Tomato Ragu	45
112.	Minted Lamb with A Couscous Salad	45
113.	Garbanzo Kale Curry	46
114.	Buckwheat Kasha with Mushrooms and Onions	46
115.	Sirtfood Cauliflower Couscous & Turkey Steak	46
116.	Turkey Escalope with Cauliflower Couscous	47
117.	Tomato & Goat's Cheese Pizza	47
118.	Roast Duck Legs with Red Wine Sauce	47
119.	Arugula-Stuffed Steak	48
120.	Beef Stroganoff French Bread Toast	48
121.	Beef Burritos	49
122.	Meatballs with Eggplant	49
123.	Slow-Cooked Lemon Chicken	49
124.	Smothered Pork Chops and Sautéed Greens	50
125.	Pasta with Cheesy Meat Sauce	50
126.	Aromatic Herbed Rice	51
127.	Herb-Crusted Roast Leg of Lamb	51
128.	Baked Potatoes with Spicy Chickpea	51
129.	Buckwheat with Red Onion Dal	52
130.	Aromatic Chicken	52
131.	Fragrant Asian hotpot-Sirtfood	53
132.	Buckwheat Bean Risotto	53
133.	Butterbean and Vegetable	53
134.	Lemon Paprika Chicken with Vegetable	54
135.	Spicy Ras-El-Hanout Dressing	54
136.	Broccoli & Mushroom Chicken	54
137.	Beef with Kale & Carrot	54
138.	Lamb Chops with Kale	55
139.	Chickpea with Swiss Chard	55
140.	Tofu & Broccoli Curry	55
141.	Chicken & Veggies with Buckwheat Noodles	56
142.	Veggie Burgers	56
143.	Kale with Pine Nuts	57
144.	Bok Choy & Mushroom Stir Fry	57
145.	Prawns with Asparagus	57

SIDES RECIPES 59

#	Recipe	Page
146.	Eggplant Dipped Roasted Asparagus	59
147.	Steamed Asparagus & Grilled Cauliflower Steaks	59
148.	Endive with Cheddar & Walnut Sauce	59
149.	Asian-Style Tofu Zucchini Kabobs	60
150.	Nutty Tofu Loaf	60
151.	Chili Toasted Nuts	60
152.	Creole Tofu Scramble with Kale	60
153.	Vegetable Frittata with Red Onions & Green Chilies	61
154.	Sirtfood Frittata	61
155.	Baby Arugula Stuffed Zucchini	61
156.	Celery Buckwheat Croquettes	62
157.	Creole Tempeh & Black Bean Bowls	62
158.	Spicy Broccoli Pasta	62
159.	Buckwheat Pilaf with Pine Nuts	63
160.	Buckwheat Savoy Cabbage Rolls with Tofu	63
161.	Potato and Chickpea Bake	63
162.	Kale Dhal with Buckwheat	64
163.	Braised Puy Lentils	64
164.	Chicken Chili with Buckwheat	65
165.	Chickpea and Quinoa Curry	65
166.	Vegetable Chili	66
167.	Lemon Splash Tofu	66
168.	Veggie Stuffed Peppers	66
169.	Veggie Jambalaya	66
170.	Veggie Stir Fry	67
171.	Buckwheat Pasta Salad	67
172.	Greek Salad on a Stick	67
173.	Tofu Curry	68
174.	Veggie and Buckwheat Stir	68
175.	Sweet Pepper Mix	69
176.	Cottage Cheese Veggie Salad	69
177.	Arugula and Lemon Rice	69
178.	Spring Pesto Beans	69
179.	Mung Sprouts Salsa	69
180.	Honey Chili Squash	70
181.	Salsa Bean Dip	70
182.	Roast Balsamic Vegetables	70
183.	Courgette and Tomato Risotto	70
184.	Black Bean Salsa	71
185.	Brown Basmati Rice Pilaf	71
186.	Crunchy Arugula with Apples	71
187.	Cauliflower and Carrots Dip	71
188.	Kale and Bean Casserole	71
189.	Red Coleslaw	72
190.	Balsamic Eggplant Salsa	72

SEAFOOD RECIPES 73

#	Recipe	Page
191.	Stir-Fried Prawn Noodles	73
192.	Buckwheat Noodles and Shrimp	73
193.	Prawn Arrabbiata	73
194.	Salmon with Turmeric	74
195.	Salmon Fillet Pan-Fried	74
196.	Sirt Food Miso Marinated Cod	75
197.	Smoked Salmon Omelet	75
198.	Seafood Salad	75
199.	Salmon Pasta Smoked with Chili/Arugula	76
200.	Minty Salmon Salad	76
201.	Stir-Fry Shrimp and Buckwheat	76
202.	Pan-Fried Salmon Fillet with Leafy Salad	77
203.	Miso-Marinated Baked Cod	77
204.	Superfood Salad	78
205.	Smoked Salmon Pasta	78
206.	Vietnamese Turmeric Fish with Herbs & Mango Sauce	78
207.	Salmon Sirt Super Salad	79
208.	Smoke Salmon with Egg	79
209.	Stir-Fried Greens, Sesame & Cod	79
210.	Turmeric Baked Salmon	80

VEGETABLE RECIPES 81

#	Recipe	Page
211.	Potato Carrot Salad	81
212.	High Protein Salad	81
213.	Vegan Wrap with Apples and Spicy Hummus	81
214.	Rice and Veggie Bowl	81
215.	Cucumber Tomato Chopped Salad	82
216.	Zucchini Pasta Salad	82

#	Recipe	Page
217.	Egg Avocado Salad	82
218.	Arugula Salad	83
219.	Sautéed Cabbage	83
220.	Cucumber Edamame Salad	83
221.	Garden Patch Sandwiches on Multigrain Bread	84
222.	Garden Salad Wraps	84
223.	Marinated Mushroom Wraps	84
224.	Tamari Toasted Almonds	85
225.	Peppers and Hummus	85
226.	Baby Spinach Snack	85
227.	Bacon Potato Bites	85
228.	Dill Bell Pepper Snack Bowls	86
229.	Spicy Pumpkin Seeds Bowls	86
230.	Apple and Pecans Bowls	86
231.	Zucchini Bowls	86
232.	Cheesy Mushrooms Caps	86
233.	Mozzarella Cauliflower Bars	87
234.	Garlic Lovers Hummus	87
235.	Spinach and Kale Mix	87
236.	Turmeric Carrots	87
237.	Spinach Mix	87
238.	Orange Carrots	88
239.	Zucchini Pan	88
240.	Stir-Fried Mushroom with Ginger	88
241.	Polenta Bake	88
242.	Raw Carrot and Almond Loaf	89
243.	Kale and Red Onion Dhal with Bucket Wheat	89
244.	Kale with Lemon Tahini Dressing	90
245.	Broccoli and Kale Green Soup	90
246.	Butter Bean and Vegetable Korma	91
247.	Courgette Tortilla	91
248.	Almond Butter and Alfalfa Wraps	92
249.	Buckwheat Bean and Tomato Risotto	92
250.	Vegetable Curry with Tofu	92
251.	Sirt Food Mushroom Scramble Eggs	93
252.	Green Salad Skewers	93
253.	Baked Potatoes with Spicy Chickpea Stew	93
254.	Buckwheat Garden Salad	94
255.	Cucumber, Pineapple, Parsley, And Lemon Smoothie	94
256.	Buckwheat Meatballs	94
257.	Cabbage and Buckwheat Fritters	95
258.	Buckwheat Salad with Artichokes	95
259.	Pasta with Rocket Salad and Linseed	96
260.	Sirt Yogurt	96
261.	Sirt Pita Bread	96
262.	Red Bean Sauce with Baked Potato	97
263.	Curly Kale with Sweet Potatoes	97
264.	Buckwheat Pasta with Zucchini and Cherry Tomatoes	97
265.	Pasta with Red Chicory and Walnuts	98
266.	Cabbage and Red Chicory Flan	98
267.	Red Chicory and Kale Salad	98
268.	Egg Scramble with Kale	99
269.	Buckwheat Porridge	99
270.	Eggs with Kale	99

SOUP AND STEW RECIPES — 101

#	Recipe	Page
271.	Miso Soup	101
272.	Mexican Chicken Soup	101
273.	Thai Spinach Soup	101
274.	Savoy Cabbage and Bacon Soup	102
275.	Edamame Beans Pesto Soup	102
276.	Spicy Butternut Squash and Kale Soup	103
277.	Kale Stilton Soup	103
278.	Curry Broth	103
279.	Walnut Soup	104
280.	Spicy Lentils Vegetable Soup	104
281.	Watercress Soup	104
282.	Curry and Rice Stew	105
283.	Chinese Style with Pak Choi	105
284.	Cauliflower Kale Curry	106
285.	Sirt Chicken Korma	106
286.	Cauliflower Soup	107
287.	Broccoli Soup	107
288.	Shrimp Soup	107
289.	Parmesan Tomato Soup	107
290.	Meatball Soup	108
291.	Eggplant Soup	108
292.	Lemon Lamb Soup	108
293.	Mushroom and Cheese Soup	109
294.	Eggplant Stew	109
295.	Leeks Soup	110
296.	Pea Stew	110
297.	Chicken Leek Soup	110
298.	Carrot Soup	110
299.	Chickpeas Stew	111
300.	Green Beans Stew	111

VEGAN RECIPES — 112

#	Recipe	Page
301.	Walnut Chocolate Cupcakes	112
302.	Sirtfood Kale Smoothie	112
303.	Fruity Matcha Smoothie	112
304.	Fresh SirtFruit Compote	112
305.	Spicy Sirtfood Ricotta	112
306.	Sirtfood Baked Potatoes	113
307.	Spicy Quinoa with Kale	113
308.	Mediterranean Sirtfood Quinoa	113
309.	Eggplant and Potatoes in Red Wine	114
310.	Potatoes with Onion Rings in Red Wine	114
311.	Sweet Potatoes with Grilled Tofu and Mushrooms	114
312.	Buckwheat Stew	115
313.	Sirtfood Curry	115
314.	Onion Mushroom Salsa	115
315.	Sirtfood Tofu Sesame Salad	116

SALAD RECIPES — 117

#	Recipe	Page
316.	Cucumber Rolls on Cauliflower Salad	117
317.	Sweet Potato Salad with Spinach, Apple and Quinoa	117
318.	Avocado and Mozzarella Salad Bowl	118
319.	Chicory and Orange Salad	118
320.	Mango and Avocado Salad with Watercress	118
321.	Coconut Pancakes with Kiwi Salad	119
322.	Salads with Oranges	119
323.	Autumn Salad	119
324.	Creamy Salmon Salad	120
325.	May Beet Salad with Cucumber	120
326.	Lentil Salad with Spinach, Rhubarb and Asparagus	121
327.	Spicy Onion Meatballs with Potato Salad	121
328.	Tomato and Zucchini Salad with Feta	122

No.	Recipe	Page
329.	Cucumber and Radish Salad with Feta	122
330.	Baked Salmon Salad with Creamy Mint Dressing	122
331.	Green Juice Salad	123
332.	Strawberry Buckwheat Salad	123
333.	Salmon Salad	123
334.	Chicken Sirtfood Salad	123
335.	Sirtfood Pesto Buckwheat Salad	124
336.	Kale Tofu Stir Fry	124
337.	Greek Stuffed Portobello Mushrooms	125
338.	Turmeric Sautéed Greens	125
339.	Sautéed Collard Greens	125
340.	Brussels Sprouts With Turmeric and Mustard Seeds	125
341.	Sirt Salad	126
342.	Buckwheat Tabbouleh and Strawberry	126
343.	Smoked-Tender Salmon Sirt Salad	126
344.	Coronation Chicken Salad	127
345.	Salad Buckwheat Pasta	127
346.	Cucumber & Onion Salad	127
347.	Citrus Fruit Salad	127
348.	Mixed Berries Salad	128
349.	Orange and Beet Salad	128
350.	Strawberry, Apple & Arugula Salad	128
351.	Shrimp Salad	128
352.	Smoked Salmon Sirt Salad	128
353.	Waldorf Salad	129
354.	Brown Rice Salad with Octopus	129
355.	Exotic Rice Salad	129
356.	Light Tuna and Bread Salad	130
357.	Spicy Avocado Salad	130
358.	Hot Chicory & Nut Salad	130
359.	Tuna, Egg & Caper Salad	131
360.	Nutty Fruit Granola	131

DESSERT RECIPES 132

No.	Recipe	Page
361.	Snow-Flakes	132
362.	Lemon Ricotta Cookies with Lemon Glaze	132
363.	Homemade Marshmallow Fluff	132
364.	Banana Ice-Cream	133
365.	Perfect Little Snack Balls	133
366.	Loaded Chocolate Pretzel Cookies	133
367.	Mascarpone Cheesecake with Almond Crust	133
368.	Marshmallow Popcorn Balls	134
369.	Homemade Ice-Cream Drumsticks	134
370.	Ultimate Chocolate Chip Cookie Fudge Brownie Bar	134
371.	Matcha Apple & Green Juice	135
372.	Apple, Cucumber & Celery Juice	135
373.	Lemony Apple & Kale Juice	135
374.	Watermelon Juice	135
375.	Apple Muffins	136
376.	Dark Chocolate Terrine	136
377.	Dark Chocolate Oatmeal	137
378.	Dark Chocolate Nut Bars	137
379.	Dark Chocolate Martini	138
380.	Dark Chocolate Brownies	138
381.	Dark-Choco Mousse	138
382.	Strawberry Buckwheat Pancakes	139
383.	Strawberry & Nut Granola	139
384.	Chilled Strawberry & Walnut Porridge	139
385.	Sweet Oatmeal	140
386.	Watergate Salad Recipe	140
387.	Moroccan Leeks Snack	140
388.	Strawberry Pretzel Salad	140
389.	Sheet Pan Apple Pie Bake	141
390.	Heaven on Earth Cake	141
391.	Strawberry Upside-Down Cake	142
392.	Lemon Blueberry Poke Cake	142
393.	Easy No-Churn Funfetti Ice Cream Cake	142
394.	Lemon Tofu Cheesecake	143
395.	Blueberry Walnut Crisp	143
396.	Red Wine Poached Pears	143
397.	Dark Chocolate Walnut No-Bake Cookies	144
398.	No-Bake Triple Berry Mini Tarts	144
399.	Mocha Buckwheat Pudding	145
400.	Loaded Chocolate Fudge	145

CONCLUSION 146

INTRODUCTION

The Sirtfood Diet is named after two ingredients that form the key to maintaining a healthy weight. Sirtfoods – as they are named – are natural plant foods that contain compounds called Sirtuins which are believed to serve as 'longevity proteins', as they work within our body in a similar way as the protein that slows down the ageing process of animals. Researchers have learnt that foods rich in Sirtuins increase the likelihood of a man or woman living longer, therefore they promote a longer and happier life. As of today, there are seven known Sirtuins described in nature – these being Sirt1, Sirt2, Sirt3, Sirt4, Sirt5, Sirt6 and Sirt7. Sirtuin 1 (Sirt1) is active in the mammalian brain, liver, intestine, kidney, and heart, having the ability to regulate the body's metabolism and control energy expenditure. Sirt1 was discovered in yeast cells in 1999 and further studies conducted in mice have since revealed that Sirt1 increases the activity of other genes, thus encouraging the breakdown of body fat and an increase in the production of good cholesterol.

Sirtfood Diet – This is the only book on the market written bout sirtfoods. To view the full story, click the images above or click here

It is thought that sirtfoods are essentially a key part of the Mediterranean diet, which was recently found to be the healthiest diet in the world. Mediterranean diet foods include a number of fruits and vegetables that are rich in these longevity proteins, resulting in their energising activity on the body. More particularly, sirtfoods are thought to prolong life by reducing the likelihood of some of the diet-related killers like heart disease and prostate cancer. Sirtuins are the same longevity proteins inside yeast cells that are also found in the Greek yogurt that is included in the Sirtfood Diet. Studies that have been carried out on mice and men have found that sirtfoods increase the length of life, because Sirt1 delays the onset of various age-related diseases. The thought is that sirtfoods act as internal 'longevity proteins.' Sirt1 works by fusing to DNA, which then produces proteins that translate into healthy cells that encode longer life. The 'yoga of eating' means that the Sirtfood Diet includes a wide variety of healthy foods, which should help to form a complete natural system. Instead of following a fad diet, this book is the perfect way to start a new, long and healthy life. This book was written with the use of The American Journal of Clinical Nutrition research, as a reference of natural weight loss and longevity factors.

APPETIZER AND SNACK RECIPES

Fruit Salad
Preparation Time: 13 minutes
Cooking Time: 0 minutes
Servings: 1
Ingredients:
- ½ cup crisply made green tea
- 1 teaspoon nectar One orange, split
- One apple, cored and generally cleaved
- Ten red seedless grapes
- Ten blueberries

Directions:
1. Stir the nectar into a large portion of some green tea. At the point when broken up, include the juice of a large part of the orange. Leave to cool.
2. Chop the other portion of the orange and spot in a bowl together with the hacked apple, blueberries and grapes. Transfer over the cooled tea and leave to soak for a couple of moments before serving.

Nutrition: 157 Calories 1g Fiber 0.5g Protein

Golden Turmeric Latte
Preparation Time: 3 minutes
Cooking Time: 7 minutes
Servings: 3
Ingredients:
- 3 cups of coconut milk
- One teaspoon turmeric powder
- One teaspoon cinnamon powder
- One teaspoon crude nectar

Directions:
1. Spot of dark pepper (expands retention)
2. Modest bit of new stripped ginger root
3. Place of cayenne pepper (discretionary)
4. Mix all fixings in a fast blender until smooth.
5. Fill a little container and warmth for 4 minutes over medium heat until hot however not bubbling.

Nutrition: 50 Calories 98g carbohydrates 2.7g Fat

The Sirt Juice
Preparation Time: 7 minutes
Cooking Time: 0 minute
Servings: 2
Ingredients:
- Two huge bunches (75g) kale
- A huge bunch (30g) rocket
- A tiny bunch (5g) level leaf parsley
- A small bunch (5g) lovage leaves (discretionary)
- 2–3 huge stalks (150g) green celery, including its leaves
- ½ medium green apple
- Juice of ½ lemon
- ½ level teaspoon Matcha green tea

Directions:
1. Blend the greens (kale, rocket, parsley and lovage, on the off chance that was utilizing), at that point juice them.
2. Presently squeeze the celery and apple. You can strip the lemon and put it through the juicer also, however, we think that it's a lot simpler just to crush the lemon by hand into the juice.
3. Pour a limited quantity of the juice into a glass, at that point include the Matcha and mix enthusiastically with a fork or teaspoon.
4. Give it a last mix; at that point, your juice is prepared to drink. Don't hesitate to top up with plain water, as indicated by taste.

Nutrition: 75 Calories 0.6g Fat 0.4g Protein

Kale Pesto Hummus
Preparation Time: 12 minutes
Cooking Time: 7 minutes
Servings: 12
Ingredients:
- Chickpeas, drained and liquid reserved – 15 ounces
- Reserved chickpea liquid - .25 cup
- Sea salt - .5 teaspoon
- Tahini paste - .5 cup
- Garlic, minced – 2 cloves
- Lemon juice – 2.5 s
- Extra virgin olive oil - .33 cup
- Black pepper, ground - .5 teaspoon
- Kale, chopped and leaves packed – 2 cups
- Pine nuts – 2 s
- Basil leaves, packed – 1.25 cups
- Garlic, minced – 4 cloves
- Extra virgin olive oil - .25 cup

Directions:
1. Into a food processor add the basil, kale, pine nuts, and four cloves of minced garlic. Pulse until the leaves and garlic are finely chopped.
2. Pour in the olive oil, and once again pulse until smooth. Remove the pesto from the bowl of the food processor and set aside.
3. Into the empty food processor add the remaining ingredients to assemble the hummus, pulsing until creamy. Add in the prepared pesto, and pulse just until the two are combined.
4. Transfer the pesto hummus to a serving bowl or store in the fridge.

Nutrition: 194 Calories 2.2g Fat 5.6g Protein

■ Parsley Hummus

Preparation Time: 6 minutes
Cooking Time: 7 minutes
Servings: 6
Ingredients:
- Chickpeas, drained and rinsed – 15 ounces
- Curly parsley, stems removed – 1 cup
- Sea salt – .5 teaspoon
- Soy milk, unsweetened - .5 cup
- Extra virgin olive oil – 3 teaspoons
- Lime juice – 1 s
- Red pepper flakes -.5 teaspoons
- Black pepper, ground - .25 teaspoon
- Pine nuts – 2 s
- Sesame seeds, toasted – 2 s

Directions:
1. In the food processor blend parsley and toasted sesame. Pour extra virgin olive oil in while you continue to pulse, until it is smooth.
2. Add the chickpeas, lime juice, and seasonings to the food processor and pulse while slowly adding in the soy milk. Continue to pulse the parsley hummus until it is smooth and creamy.
3. Adjust the seasonings to your preference and then serve or refrigerate the hummus.

Nutrition: 107 Calories 4.5g Fat 8.6g Protein

■ Edamame Hummus

Preparation Time: 8 minutes
Cooking Time: 0 minutes
Servings: 10
Ingredients:
- Edamame, cooked and shelled – 2 cups
- Sea salt – 1 teaspoon
- Extra virgin olive oil – 1
- Tahini paste - .25 cup
- Lemon juice - .25 cup
- Garlic, minced – 3 cloves
- Black pepper, ground - .25 teaspoon

Directions:
1. Add the cooked edamame and remaining ingredients to a blender or food processor and mix on high until it forms a creamy and completely smooth mixture. Taste it and adjust the seasonings to your preference.
2. Serve the hummus immediately with your favorite vegetables or store in the fridge.

Nutrition: 88 Calories 3.8g carbohydrates 2.6g Protein

■ Edamame Guacamole

Preparation Time: 8 minutes
Cooking Time: 0 minutes
Servings: 6
Ingredients:
- Edamame, cooked and shelled – 1 cup
- Avocado, pitted and halved – 1
- Red onion, diced - .5 cup
- Cilantro, chopped - .25 cup
- Jalapeno, minced – 1
- Garlic, minced – 2 cloves
- Lime juice – 2 s Water – 3 s
- Lime zest - .5 teaspoon
- Roma tomato, diced – 2
- Cumin - .125 teaspoon
- Sea salt - .5 teaspoon

Directions:
1. Using food processor add all of the ingredients, except for the diced tomato, onion, and jalapeno. Blend the tomato mixture on high speed until it is smooth and creamy, making sure that the edamame has been completely blended.
2. Adjust the seasoning to your preference and then transfer the guacamole to a serving bowl. Stir in the tomato, onion, and jalapeno. Place the bowl in the fridge, allowing it to chill for at least thirty minutes before serving.

Nutrition: 100 Calories 6.6g Fat 45g Protein

Eggplant Fries with Fresh Aioli

Preparation Time: 16 minutes
Cooking Time: 27 minutes
Servings: 4

Ingredients:
- Eggplants – 2
- Black pepper, ground - .25 teaspoon
- Extra virgin olive oil – 2 s
- Cornstarch – 1
- Basil, dried – 1 teaspoon
- Garlic powder - .25 teaspoon
- Sea salt - .5 teaspoon
- Mayonnaise, made with olive oil - .5 cup
- Garlic, minced – 1 teaspoon
- Basil, fresh, chopped – 1
- Lemon juice – 1 teaspoon
- Chipotle, ground - .5 teaspoon
- Sea salt - .25 teaspoon

Directions:
1. Begin by preheating your oven to Fahrenheit four-hundred and twenty-five degrees. Place a wire cooking/cooling rack on a baking sheet.
2. Remove the peel from the eggplants and then slice them into rounds, each about three-quarters of an inch thick. Slice the rounds into wedges one inch in width.
3. Add the eggplant wedges to a large bowl and toss them with the olive oil. Once coated, add the pepper, cornstarch, dried basil, garlic powder, and sea salt, tossing until evenly coated.
4. Arrange the eggplant wedges on top of the wire rack and set the baking sheet in the oven, allowing the fries to cook for fifteen to twenty minutes.
5. Meanwhile, prepare the aioli. To do this, add the remaining ingredients into a small bowl and whisk them together to combine. Cover the bowl of aioli and allow it to chill it in the fridge until the fries are ready to be served.
6. Remove the fries from the oven immediately upon baking, or allow them to cook under the broiler for an additional three to four minutes for extra crispy fries. Serve immediately with the aioli.

Nutrition: 243 Calories 0.5g Fat 5.3g Protein

Eggplant Caponata

Preparation Time: 13 minutes
Cooking time: 25 minutes
Servings: 4

Ingredients:
- Eggplant, sliced into 1.5-inch cubes – 1 pound
- Bell pepper, diced – 1
- Green and black olives, chopped - .5 cup
- Capers - .25 cup
- Sea salt – 1 teaspoon
- Garlic, minced – 4
- Red onion, diced – 1
- Diced tomatoes – 15 ounces
- Extra virgin olive oil – 4 s, divided
- Black pepper, ground - .25 teaspoon
- Parsley, chopped - .25 cup

Directions:
1. Preheat your oven to Fahrenheit four-hundred degrees and line a baking sheet with kitchen parchment.
2. Toss the eggplant cubes in half of the olive oil and then arrange them on the baking sheet, sprinkling the sea salt over the top. Allow the eggplant to roast until tender, about twenty minutes.
3. Meanwhile, add the remaining olive oil into a large skillet along with the red onions, bell pepper, diced tomatoes, and garlic. Sautee the vegetables until tender, about ten minutes.
4. Add the roasted eggplant, capers, olives, and black pepper to the skillet, continuing to cook together for five minutes so that the flavors meld.
5. Remove the skillet from the heat, top it off with parsley, and serve it with crusty toast.

Nutrition: 209 Calories 2.3g Fat 0.3g Protein

Buckwheat Crackers

Preparation Time: 8 minutes
Cooking Time: 1 hour
Servings: 12

Ingredients:
- Buckwheat groats – 2 cups
- Flaxseeds, ground - .75 cup

- Sesame seeds - .33 cup
- Sweet potatoes, medium, grated – 2
- Extra virgin olive oil – .33 cup
- Water – 1 cup
- Sea salt – 1 teaspoon

Directions:
1. Soak the buckwheat groats in water for at least four hours before preparing the crackers. Once done soaking, drain off the water.
2. Preheat the oven to a temperature of Fahrenheit three-hundred and fifty degrees, prepare a baking sheet, and set aside some kitchen parchment and plastic wrap.
3. In a kitchen bowl, combine the ground flaxseeds with the warm water, allowing the seeds to absorb the water and form a substance similar to gelatin. Add the buckwheat groats and other remaining ingredients.
4. Spread the cracker dough onto a sheet of kitchen parchment and cover it with a sheet of plastic wrap. Use a rolling pen on top of the plastic wrap (so that it doesn't stick) and roll out the buckwheat cracker dough until it is thin.
5. Peel the plastic wrap off of the crackers and transfer the dough-coated sheet of kitchen parchment to the prepared baking sheet. Allow it to partially bake for fifteen minutes and then remove the tray from the oven.
6. Reduce the oven temperature to Fahrenheit three-hundred degrees. Use a pizza cutter and slice the crackers into squares, approximately two inches in width. Return the crackers to the oven until they are crispy and dry, about thirty-five to forty minutes.
7. Remove the crackers from the oven, allowing them to cool completely before storing them in an air-tight container.

Nutrition: 158 Calories 3.8g Fat 3.4g Protein

Matcha Protein Bites

Preparation Time: 18 minutes
Cooking Time: 70 minutes
Servings: 12

Ingredients:
- Almond butter - .25 cup
- Matcha powder – 2 teaspoons
- Soy protein isolate – 1 ounce
- Rolled oats - .5 cup
- Chia seeds – 1
- Coconut oil – 2 teaspoons
- Honey – 1
- Sea salt - .125 teaspoon

Directions:
1. Using food processor, process all of the Matcha protein bite ingredients until it forms a mixture similar to wet sand, that will stick together when squished between your fingers.
2. Divide the mixture into twelve equal portions. Form into balls.
3. Chill the bites in the fridge for up to two weeks.

Nutrition: 164 Calories 4.7g Fat 4.5g Protein

Chocolate-Covered Strawberry Trail Mix

Preparation Time: 7 minutes
Cooking Time: 0 minutes
Servings: 10

Ingredients:
- Freeze-dried strawberries – 1 cup
- Dark chocolate chunks - .66 cup
- Walnuts, roasted – 1 cup
- Almonds, roasted - .25 cup
- Cashews, roasted - .25 cup

Directions:
1. Mix together all of the trail mix ingredients in a bowl, and then store it in a large glass jar or divide each serving into its own transportable plastic bag. Store for up to one month.

Nutrition: 164 Calories 3.2g Fat 2.2g Protein

Moroccan Spiced Eggs

Preparation Time: 71 minutes
Cooking Time: 42 minutes
Servings: 2

Ingredients:
- 1 tablespoon olive oil
- One shallot, stripped and finely hacked
- One red (chime) pepper, deseeded and finely hacked
- One garlic clove, stripped and finely hacked

- One courgette (zucchini), stripped and finely hacked
- 1 tablespoon tomato puree (glue)
- ½ teaspoon gentle stew powder
- ¼ teaspoon ground cinnamon
- ¼ teaspoon ground cumin
- ½ teaspoon salt
- 400g can hacked tomatoes
- 400g may chickpeas in water
- A little bunch of level leaf parsley cleaved
- Four medium eggs at room temperature

Directions:
1. Heat the oil in a pan, include the shallot and red (ringer) pepper and fry delicately for 5 minutes. At that point include the garlic and courgette (zucchini) and cook for one more moment or two. Include the tomato puree (glue), flavors and salt and mix through.
2. Add the cleaved tomatoes and chickpeas (dousing alcohol and all) and increment the warmth to medium. With the top of the dish, stew the sauce for 30 minutes – ensure it is delicately rising all through and permit it to lessen in volume by around 33%.
3. Remove from the warmth and mix in the cleaved parsley.
4. Preheat the grill to 200C/180C fan/350F.
5. When you are prepared to cook the eggs, bring the tomato sauce up to a delicate stew and move to a little broiler confirmation dish.
6. Crack the eggs on the dish and lower them delicately into the stew. Spread with thwart and prepare in the grill for 10-15 minutes. Serve the blend in unique dishes with the eggs coasting on the top.

Nutrition: 116 Calorie 6.97g Protein 5.22g Fat

Exquisite Turmeric Pancakes with Lemon Yogurt Sauce

Preparation Time: 43 minutes
Cooking Time: 18 minutes
Servings: 8 hotcakes

Ingredients:
For Yogurt Sauce
- 1 cup Greek yogurt
- 1 garlic clove
- 2 tablespoons lemon juice
- ¼ tsp. ground turmeric
- 10 crisp mint leaves
- 2 teaspoons lemon wedges

For Pancakes
- 2 tsp. ground turmeric
- 1½ tsp. ground cumin
- 1 tsp. salt
- 1 tsp. ground coriander
- ½ tsp. garlic powder
- ½ teaspoon naturally ground dark pepper
- 1 head broccoli, cut into florets
- 3 enormous eggs, gently beaten
- 2 tablespoons plain unsweetened almond milk
- 1 cup almond flour
- 4 teaspoons coconut oil

Directions:
1. Make the yogurt sauce. Join the yogurt, garlic, lemon juice, turmeric, mint and pizzazz in a bowl. Taste and enjoy with more lemon juice, if possible. Keep in a safe spot or freeze until prepared to serve.
2. Make the flapjacks. In a little bowl, join the turmeric, cumin, salt, coriander, garlic and pepper.
3. Spot the broccoli in a nourishment processor, and heartbeat until the florets are separated into little pieces. Move the broccoli to an enormous bowl and include the eggs, almond milk, and almond flour. Mix in the flavor blend and consolidate well.
4. Cook 1 teaspoon of the coconut oil in a nonstick dish over medium-low heat. Empty ¼ cup player into the skillet. Cook the hotcake until little air pockets start to show up superficially and the base is brilliant darker, 2 to 3 minutes. Flip over and cook the hotcake for 2 to 3 minutes more. To keep warm, move the cooked hotcakes to a stove safe dish and spot in a 200°F oven.
5. Keep making the staying 3 hotcakes, utilizing the rest of the oil and player.

Nutrition: 262 Calories 11.7g Protein 19.2g Fat

Sirt Chili Con Carne

Preparation Time: 82 minutes
Cooking Time: 63 minutes
Servings: 4
Ingredients:
- 1 red onion, finely cleaved
- 3 garlic cloves, finely cleaved
- 2 chilies, finely hacked
- 1 tablespoon additional virgin olive oil
- 1 tablespoon ground cumin
- 1 tablespoon ground turmeric
- 400g lean minced hamburger
- 150ml red wine
- 1 red pepper, cored
- 2 x 400g tins cleaved tomatoes
- 1 tablespoon tomato purée
- 1 tablespoon cocoa powder
- 150g tinned kidney beans
- 300ml hamburger stock
- 5g coriander, cleaved
- 5g parsley, cleaved
- 160g buckwheat

Directions:
1. Fry onion, garlic and bean stew in the oil at medium heat for 2 minutes.
2. Include the minced hamburger and dark colored at high heat. Pour in the red wine
3. Mix red pepper, tomatoes, tomato purée, cocoa, kidney beans and stock and keep aside for 1 hour.
4. Once thick, mix in the hacked herbs. Cook the buckwheat then serve with the stew.

Nutrition: 346 Calories 14.11g Protein 11.37g Fat

Med-Style Olives

Preparation Time: 13 minutes
Cooking Time: 9 minutes
Servings: 6
Ingredients:
- One pinch of salt One pinch of black pepper
- 1 ½ tablespoon of coriander seeds
- One tablespoon of extra-virgin olive oil
- One lemon
- 7 oz. of kalamata olives
- 7 oz. of green queen olives

Directions:
1. Pound the coriander seeds and set aside.
2. Slice long, thin of lemon rind and mix with both the green queen and kalamata olives.
3. Pour lemon juice on top of the olives and mix olive oil.
4. Add the salt, pepper, and coriander seeds, then stir and serve.

Nutrition: 477 Calories 9g Fat 35g Protein

Crispy Chickpeas

Preparation Time: 14 minutes
Cooking Time: 38 minutes
Servings: 6
Ingredients:
- One pinch of salt
- One pinch of black pepper
- One pinch of garlic powder
- One teaspoon of dried oregano
- Two tablespoons of extra-virgin olive oil
- juice of 1 lemon
- Two teaspoons of red wine vinegar
- 2 15 oz. canned chickpeas

Directions:
1. Preheat your oven to 42 5 F and place a sheet of parchment paper onto a baking tray.
2. Drain and rinse the chickpeas, then pour them onto the baking tray. Spread equally. Roast for 11 minutes. Pull it out then shake. Cook again for 10 minutes. Once roasted, put aside.
3. Mix remaining ingredients and stir in roasted chickpeas. Put the chickpeas back to the oven and roast for 11 minutes. Pull it out, cool, then serve.

Nutrition: 323 Calories 15.6g fat 10.4g Protein

Honey Chili Nuts

Preparation Time: 13 minutes
Cooking Time: 31 minutes
Servings: 4
Ingredients:
- 5oz walnuts
- 5oz pecan nuts
- 2oz softened butter
- 1 tablespoon honey
- ½ bird's-eye chili, very finely chopped and deseeded

Directions:

1. Preheat the oven to 180C/360F. Combine the butter, honey, and chili in a bowl, then add the nuts and stir them well.
2. Lay out the nuts in a lined baking sheet and roast them in the oven for 10 minutes, stirring once halfway through. Pull out from the oven and cool before eating.

Nutrition: 65g Calories 0.5g Fat 2g Protein

Cauliflower Nachos

Preparation Time: 7 minutes
Cooking Time: 33 minutes
Servings: 2

Ingredients:
- 2 tablespoons extra virgin olive oil
- ½ teaspoon onion powder
- ½ teaspoon turmeric
- ½ teaspoon ground cumin
- 1 medium head cauliflower
- ¾ cup shredded cheddar cheese
- ½ cup tomato, diced
- ¼ cup red bell pepper, diced
- ¼ cup red onion, diced
- ½ Bird's Eye chili pepper, finely diced
- ¼ cup parsley, finely diced
- Pinch of salt

Directions:
1. Preheat oven to 400 ° F.
2. Mix onion powder, cumin, turmeric, and olive oil. Core cauliflower and slice into ½" thick rounds. Coat the cauliflower with the olive oil mixture and bake for 15 – 20 minutes.
3. Top with shredded cheese & bake for an additional 3 – 5 minutes, until cheese is melted. In a bowl, combine tomatoes, bell pepper, onion, chili, and parsley with a pinch of salt.
4. Top cooked cauliflower with salsa and serve.

Nutrition: 195 Calories 5g Fat 3.6g Protein

Cheesy Cauliflower Bars

Preparation Time: 14 minutes
Cooking Time: 39 minutes
Servings: 1

Ingredients:
- ½ cauliflower head, riced
- 1/3 cup low-fat mozzarella cheese, shredded
- ¼ cup egg whites
- 1 teaspoon Italian dressing, low fat
- Pepper to taste

Directions:
1. Lay out cauliflower rice over a lined baking sheet. Preheat your oven to 375 degrees F. Roast for 20 minutes. Transfer to a bowl and spread pepper, cheese, seasoning, egg whites, and stir well.
2. Spread in a rectangular pan and press. Situate in an oven and cook for 20 minutes. Serve and enjoy!

Nutrition: 90 Calories 4g Fat 4g Protein

Walnut and Date Bites

Preparation Time: 7 minutes
Cooking Time: 0 minutes
Servings: 1

Ingredients:
- 3 walnut halves
- 3 pitted Medjool dates
- the ground cinnamon, to taste

Directions:
1. Cut each walnut carefully into three slices, and do the same with dates. Put a slice of walnut, brush with cinnamon, and serve.

Nutrition: 78 Calories 7g Fat 1.5g Protein

Sirt Energy Balls

Preparation Time: 9 minutes
Cooking Time: 11 minutes
Servings: 5

Ingredients:
- 1 cup old fashion ginger, dried
- 1/4 cup quinoa cooked
- 1/4 cup shredded unsweetened coconut
- 1/3 cup dried cranberry/raisin blend
- 1/3 cup dark chocolate chips
- 1/4 cup slivered almonds
- 1 Tbsp reduced-fat peanut butter

Directions:
1. Cook quinoa in orange juice. Boil and simmer for 4 minutes. Let cool. Combine chilled quinoa and the remaining ingredients into a bowl.
2. With wet hands and combine ingredients and roll in golden ball sized chunks.
3. Set at a Tupperware and chill until the firm.

Nutrition: 80 Calories 7g Fat 2.5g Protein

Celery and Raisins Snack Salad

Preparation Time: 16 minutes
Cooking Time: 0 minutes
Servings: 4

Ingredients:

- ½ cup raisins
- 4 cups celery, sliced
- ¼ cup parsley, chopped
- ½ cup walnuts, chopped
- Juice of ½ lemon
- 2 tbsp. extra virgin olive oil
- Salt and black pepper to the taste

Directions:

1. In a salad bowl, mix celery with raisins, walnuts, parsley, lemon juice, oil, and black pepper, toss, divide into small cups and serve as a snack.

Nutrition: 120 Calories 1g Fat 5g Protein

Yogurt & Fruit Jam Parfait

Preparation Time: 6 minutes
Cooking Time: 5 minutes
Servings: 6

Ingredients:

- 3 cups Mixed Berries
- 1 tbsp. Lemon Juice
- 7/8 cup Honey
- 2 tsp. Fruit Pectin
- 1 cup Granola
- 3 cups Greek Yoghurt

Directions:

1. For making this healthy jam, you need to place the mixed berries, honey, lemon juice, and pectin in the blender pitcher.
2. Next, pulse the mixture 3 to 4 times and then press the 'sauce/ dip' button.
3. Now, transfer the jam to a safe heat container and then place it in the refrigerator for 2 to 3 hours.
4. Once the jam is chilled, layer 1/3 cup of the Greek Yoghurt into the bottom of the parfait glass.
5. After that, spoon in a jam into it and then add the granola.
6. Serve immediately.

Nutrition: 154 calories 4g fat 9g protein

Lemon Ricotta Cookies

Preparation Time: 19 minutes
Cooking Time: 17 Minutes
Servings: 12

Ingredients:

- 2 1/2 cups all-purpose flour
- 1 tsp. baking powder
- 1 tsp. salt
- 1 tbsp. unsalted butter softened
- 2 cups of sugar
- 2 capsules
- 1 teaspoon (15-ounce) container whole-milk ricotta cheese
- 3 tbsp. lemon juice
- 1 lemon

Glaze:

- 11/2 cups powdered sugar
- 3 tbsp. lemon juice
- 1 lemon

Directions:

1. Pre heat the oven to 375 degrees F.
2. In a medium bowl combine the flour, baking powder, and salt. Set-aside.
3. Incorporate butter and the sugar levels. Scourge sugar and butter for three minutes. Pour eggs 1 at a time, while beating.
4. Beat ricotta cheese, lemon juice and lemon zest. Mix in the dry skin.
5. Line two baking sheets with parchment paper. Spoon the dough (approximately 2 tablespoons of each cookie) on the baking sheets. Bake for 14 minutes. Pull it out then set aside for 21 minutes.
6. Combine the powdered sugar lemon juice and lemon peel then stir. Scoop about 1/2-tsp on each cookie and press. Allow glaze harden for approximately two hours. Pack the biscuits to a decorative jar.

Nutrition: 24.5g Carbohydrates 13.4g Protein 2g Fat

Matcha Mochi

Preparation Time: 2 minutes
Cooking Time: 19 Minutes
Servings: 2

Ingredients:

- 1 cup Superfine White Rice Flour
- 1 cup of coconut milk
- 2 tablespoons Matcha powder

- 1/2 cup sugar
- 2 tablespoons butter melted
- 1 teaspoon baking powder

Directions:
1. Preheat the oven to 325. Spray baking dish with non-stick spray. Mix all dry ingredients, including sugar.
2. Whisk to blend. Add melted butter and coconut milk. Stir well. Put into a baking dish. Bake for 20 minutes.

Nutrition: 170 Calories 4.3g Fat 4.9g Protein

Blueberry Muffins

Preparation Time: 14 minutes
Cooking Time: 28 Minutes
Servings: 10

Ingredients:
- 1 cup Fresh blueberries
- 2 Tbsp Melted coconut oil
- 2 Tbsp Maple syrup
- 2 Eggs
- 5 cup Almond milk
- A pinch of Salt
- tsp Baking powder
- ¼ cup Arrowroot starch
- 1 cup Buckwheat flour

Directions:
1. Set oven to 350 degrees. Prepare a muffin tin.
2. Bring out a bowl and add the salt, baking powder, arrowroot starch, and buckwheat flour.
3. Using a new bowl, mix the eggs, milk, oil, and syrup together. Beat them together until well combined. Add in the flour mixture and then fold in the blueberries.
4. Move to the muffin tins and then add into the oven. Bake for 25 minutes. When these are done, take them out to cool and then serve.

Nutrition: 391 calories 19g fats 13g protein

Brownie Bites

Preparation Time: 2 hours
Cooking Time: 0 minutes
Servings: 12

Ingredients:
- 2 ½ cups whole walnuts
- ¼ cup almonds
- 2 ½ cups Medjool0dates
- 1 cup cacao powder
- 1 teaspoon vanilla extract
- ¼ tsp. sea salt

Directions:
1. Blend all the ingredients using food processor.
2. Form into balls and situate on a baking sheet and freeze for 30 minutes.

Nutrition: 110 Calories 2.8g Fat 5g Protein

Mascarpone Cheesecake

Preparation Time: 12 minutes
Cooking Time: 23 minutes
Servings: 3

Ingredients:

Crust
- 1/2 cup slivered almonds
- 8 tsp. -- or 2/3 cup graham cracker crumbs
- 2 tbsp. sugar
- 1 tbsp. salted butter melted

Filling
- 1 (8-ounce) packages cream cheese, room temperature
- 1 (8-ounce) container mascarpone cheese, room temperature
- 3/4 cup sugar
- 1 tsp. fresh lemon juice (or imitation lemon-juice)
- 1 tsp. vanilla infusion
- 2 large eggs, room temperature

Directions:
1. For the crust: prep oven at 350 degrees. Get 9-inch diameter around the pan. Pulse almonds, cracker crumbs sugar in a food processor. Mix in butter
2. Press the almond mixture on the base of the prepared pan. Bake for 2 minutes. Lower temperature to 325 degrees F.
3. For your filling: with an electric mixer, scourge cream cheese, mascarpone cheese, and sugar. Pour in the lemon juice and vanilla. Add the eggs simultaneously until combined
4. Transfer cheese mixture on the crust from the pan. Position the pan into a big skillet then put enough hot water to the roasting pan. Bake for 1 hour Transfer the cake to a stand 1 hour. Refrigerate before cheesecake is cold, at least eight hours.

5. Decorate the cake using melted chocolate

Nutrition: 5g Carbohydrates 25g Fat 5g Protein

Chocolate Berry Blend

Preparation Time: 32 minutes
Cooking Time: 0 minutes
Servings: 1

Ingredients:
- 2oz kale
- 2oz blueberries
- 2oz strawberries
- 1 banana
- 1 tablespoon 100% cocoa powder or cacao nibs
- 7 oz unsweetened soya milk

Directions:
1. Situate all of the ingredients into a blender with enough water to cover them and process until smooth.

Nutrition: 256 Calories 9g Fats 6g Protein

Monkey Trail Mix

Preparation Time: 1 hour
Cooking Time: 32 minutes
Servings: 5

Ingredients:
- One teaspoon of vanilla extract
- Three tablespoons of coconut oil
- 1/3 cup of coconut sugar
- 6 oz. of dried banana
- ½ cup of dark chocolate chips
- 1 cup of coconut flakes, unsweetened
- 1 cup of cashews, raw and unsalted
- 2 cups of walnuts, raw and unsalted

Directions:
1. Add the coconut oil, vanilla extract, coconut sugar, coconut flakes, and nuts into a crockpot.
2. Mix then cook at high for 1 hour. Stir occasionally
3. Turn the crockpot temperature to low and continue to cook for another 30 minutes.
4. Transfer the mixture out onto parchment paper and allow to dry completely.
5. Cool before adding the banana and chocolate chips.

Nutrition: 151 Calories 10g Fat 4g Protein

Granola with Quinoa

Preparation Time: 31 minutes
Cooking Time: 23 minutes
Servings: 6

Ingredients:
- One pinch of salt
- ¼ cup of maple syrup
- 3 ½ tablespoons of coconut oil
- One tablespoon coconut sugar
- 1 cup of rolled oats
- 2 cups of almonds, raw and unsalted
- ½ cup of quinoa, uncooked

Directions:
1. Prep your oven to 340 F and line a baking tray with parchment paper. In a large mixing bowl, add the salt, sugar, oats, almonds, and quinoa and set aside. Using small saucepan over medium heat, pour maple syrup and coconut oil.
2. Using a whisk, stir regularly until combined, then remove from the heat. Pour the syrup over the mixed nuts and quinoa and give it a thorough stir. Place the mixture onto the baking tray and, using a spatula, spread the ingredients evenly over the dish.
3. Bake for 20 minutes. Remove the tray, give it a shake, and return to the oven to bake for another 10 minutes.
4. Allow to cool, then serve.
5. As an alternative, you may use muscovado or brown sugar instead of coconut sugar.
6. Feel free to alternate the nut mixture depending on your tastes.

Nutrition: 241 Calories 6g Fat 15g Protein

Med-Styled Olives

Preparation Time: 17 minutes
Cooking Time: 12 minutes
Servings: 6

Ingredients:
- One pinch of salt One pinch of black pepper
- 1 ½ tablespoon of coriander seeds
- One tablespoon of extra-virgin olive oil
- One lemon
- 7 oz. of kalamata olives
- 7 oz. of green queen olives

Directions:
1. Mash the coriander seeds and set aside.
2. Cut long slices of lemon rind and situate with kalamata olives and green queen.

3. Dash with lemon juice over the top of the olives and stir olive oil.
4. Add the salt, pepper, and coriander seeds, then stir and serve.

Nutrition: 477 Calories 9g Fat 35g Protein

Roasted Chickpeas

Preparation Time: 13 minutes
Cooking Time: 41 minutes
Servings: 6
Ingredients:
- One pinch of salt One pinch of black pepper One pinch of garlic powder
- One teaspoon of dried oregano
- Two tablespoons of extra-virgin olive oil
- juice of 1 lemon
- Two teaspoons of red wine vinegar 2 15 oz. canned chickpeas

Directions:
1. Preheat your oven to 425 F and place a sheet of parchment paper onto a baking tray.
2. Drain and rinse the chickpeas, then pour them onto the baking tray. Spread evenly. Roast it for 10 minutes. Take it out, shake, then roast it again for 10 minutes. Pull it out then set aside.
3. Incorporate the rest of ingredients then mix in roasted chickpeas. Cook the chickpeas again into the oven and roast for 10 minutes. Remove, let it cool, and serve.

Nutrition: 323 Calories 16g fat 10.4g Protein

Baked Root Veg Crisps

Preparation Time: 14 minutes
Cooking Time: 29 minutes
Servings: 2
Ingredients:
- One pinch of salt
- One pinch of black pepper
- One pinch of ground cumin
- One pinch of dried thyme
- One teaspoon of garlic powder
- Two tablespoons of extra-virgin olive oil
- One parsnip, finely sliced
- One turnip, finely sliced
- One red beet, finely sliced
- One golden beet, finely sliced
- Ingredients for the dipping sauce:
- One pinch of salt
- One pinch of black pepper
- Six tablespoons of buttermilk
- 1 cup of Greek yoghurt
- One teaspoon of honey
- One teaspoon of lemon zest
- Two cloves of garlic, minced
- Two tablespoons of fresh, flat-leaf parsley, minced

Directions:
1. Combine all of the dipping sauce ingredients into a medium mixing bowl, using a whisk to ensure that the sauce is evenly combined. Set aside in the refrigerator for when needed.
2. Preheat your oven to 400 F.
3. In a small mixing bowl, combine the seasoning, herbs, and olive oil.
4. Rinse your root vegetables and dry them off using a kitchen towel. Remove all the root vegetable skins and very gently, using a mandolin slicer, slice the vegetables into thin crisps.
5. Brush each side of the crisp with the olive oil and then place onto an oven-proof wire rack. Place the wire rack onto a baking sheet and put this into the oven to bake for 20 minutes
6. Allow to cool or enjoy them warm with the sauce.

Nutrition: 457 Calories 31g Fat 12g Protein

Bubble and Squeak

Preparation Time: 1 hour
Cooking Time: 44 minutes
Servings: 3
Ingredients:
- One tablespoon butter 2 cups shredded cabbage
- One medium carrot, shredded
- ¼ cup chopped onion
- One batch The Ultimate Fauxtatoes
- ½ cup shredded Cheddar cheese

Directions:
1. Prepare the oven to 350 degrees Fahrenheit. Melt the butter in a large, massive fish and smooth the vegetables until the onion begins to turn translucent, and the cabbage becomes slightly soft.

Spray a 6-liter (1.4-litre) plate with colorless cooking spray.
2. Spread one-third of the Fauxtatoes on the bottom, then make a half layer of the cabbage mixture. Repeat the layers and finish with a Fauxtatoes layer. Cheese top. Bake for 45 minutes and strain through all layers.

Nutrition: 4g protein 2g carbohydrates 1g fiber

Thai Cucumber Salad

Preparation Time: 51 minutes
Cooking Time: 28 minutes
Servings: 8

Ingredients
- ½ small red onion
- One fresh jalapeno, seeds removed
- Three medium cucumbers
- 2 or 3 cloves fresh garlic, crushed
- Two tablespoons grated fresh ginger
- ½ cup (120 ml) rice vinegar
- ½ teaspoon salt
- ¼ teaspoon pepper
- Two tablespoons Splenda

Directions:
1. With a food processor with the S blade, place the onion and syrup solution in the food and press to crush both fine.
2. Remove the S blade and place it on the cutting disc. Rotate the cucumbers and then pass them through the processor.
3. Put onions, pumpkins, and cucumbers in a large bowl. In a separate bowl, combine the garlic, ginger, vinegar, salt, pepper, and splendor. Pour the vegetables and mix well.
4. Chill several hours before serving to get the best taste.

Nutrition: 6g carbohydrates 1g fiber 1g protein.

Mushroom Risotto

Preparation Time: 12 minutes
Cooking Time: 3 minutes.
Servings: 5

Ingredients:
- ½ head cauliflower
- Three tablespoons butter
- 1 cup sliced mushrooms
- ½ medium onion, diced
- One teaspoon minced garlic or two cloves garlic
- Two tablespoons dry vermouth
- One tablespoon chicken bouillon granule
- ¼ cup grated Parmesan cheese
- Guar or xanthan Two tablespoons chopped fresh parsley

Directions:
1. Run the cauliflower using a food processor with a razor blade. Put the cauliflower in a microwave oven, add a few tablespoons of water, and cover the microwave for 7 minutes over high heat.
2. While the cauliflower cooks, it melts
3. Put the butter in a large fish over medium heat and add the mushrooms, onion, and garlic and mix.
4. Once ready, take it out from microwave and drain it. Mix cauliflower to the fish and mix everything. Mix in Vermouth, boil, and cheese and cook for 2 to 3 minutes.
5. Simply sprinkle some guar or xanthan on the "risotto," always mixing to give it a creamy texture. Stir in parsley and serve.

Nutrition: 4g carbohydrates 1g fiber 6g protein

Cauliflower-Olive Salad

Preparation Time: 22 minutes
Cooking Time: 14 minutes.
Servings: 5

Ingredients:
- ½ head cauliflower, broken into small florets
- ½ cup diced red onion
- One can sliced ripe olives, drained
- ½ cup chopped fresh parsley
- ¼ cup lemon juice ¼ cup olive oil
- ¼ cup (mayonnaise
- ½ teaspoon salt or Vege-Sal
- About a dozen cherry tomatoes Lettuce (optional) and parsley in a bowl.

Directions:
1. Combine lemon juice, olive oil, mayonnaise, and salt in a separate bowl. Pour the vegetables and pour well.
2. When the salad is ready, cut the cherry tomatoes in half and add them to the mixture. Serve on a bed with salad, if you like, but it's great.

Nutrition: 7g carbohydrates 2g fiber 1g protein

Zucchini-Crusted Pizza

Preparation Time: 31 minutes
Cooking Time: 28 minutes
Servings: 4

Ingredients

- 3 ½ cups shredded zucchini
- Three eggs 1 ½ cup rice protein powder or soy powder
- 1½ cups shredded mozzarella, divided
- ½ cup grated Parmesan cheese
- A pinch or two of dried basil
- ½ teaspoon salt
- ¼ teaspoon pepper Oil
- 1 cup sugar-free pizza sauce
- Toppings as desired

Directions:

1. Preheat oven to 350 ° F
2. Sprinkle the pumpkin with a little salt and let stand 15-30 minutes. Put it in a straightener and press for extra moisture. Multiply the chopped pumpkin, eggs, protein powder, 2 cups of mozzarella, parmesan, basil, salt, and pepper. Spray (23 33 33 cm) pan with a non-stick cooking spray and spread the pumpkin mixture. Bake for 26 minutes
3. Wash the pumpkin peel with a little oil and cook for 5 minutes until golden. Then spread the pizza sauce and add 1 cup Mozzarella and other tops. Bake for another 25 minutes, then cut into squares and serve.

Nutrition: 14g carbohydrates 2g fiber 22g protein

Broccoli Salad

Preparation Time: 22 minutes
Cooking Time: 18 minutes
Servings: 6

Ingredients:

- ½ cup (120 ml) olive oil
- ¼ cup (60 ml) vinegar
- 1 clove garlic, crushed
- ½ teaspoon Italian seasoning herb blend
- ½ teaspoon salt or Vege-Sal
- ½ teaspoon pepper
- 4 cups frozen broccoli "cuts"

Directions:

1. Multiply the olive oil, vinegar, garlic, herbs, salt, and pepper.
2. They don't even bother you
3. Broccoli - Put it in a bowl and pour the olive oil mixture over it. Stir well and let it sit in the refrigerator for a few hours. If you think and serve it as vegetables or vegetables, mix it.

Nutrition: 7g carbohydrates 4g fiber 4g protein.

Not-Quite-Middle-Eastern Salad

Preparation Time: 22 minutes
Cooking Time: 17 minutes
Servings: 6

Ingredients:

- ½ head cauliflower
- 2/3 cup sliced stuffed olives
- Seven scallions, sliced
- 2 cups triple-washed fresh spinach, finely chopped
- One stalk celery, diced
- One small ripe tomato, finely diced
- Four tablespoons chopped parsley
- ¼ cup olive oil
- One teaspoon minced garlic or two cloves garlic, crushed
- One tablespoon red wine vinegar
- Two tablespoons mayonnaise
- Salt and pepper

Directions:

1. Run cauliflower using a food processor knife, place in a microwave oven, add a few tablespoons (30 ml) of water, cover the pan, and cook for only 5 minutes.
2. While cooking, place the olives, onions, spinach, celery, tomatoes, and parsley in a large salad bowl.
3. When the cauliflower has come out of the microwave, pour it into a rectifier and run it for a moment or two in cold water to cool.
4. Drain the cauliflower well and sprinkle with other vegetables. Add oil, garlic, vinegar and mayonnaise, and pot. Add salt and pepper to taste, bake and serve again.

Nutrition: 5g carbohydrates 2g fiber 1g protein

Apple Cinnamon Oats Bowl

Preparation Time: 12 minutes
Cooking Time: 4 minutes
Servings: 2

Ingredients:
- One green apple (skinned, cored)
- 1 cup Instant oats
- 1 scoop Soy protein isolate (chocolate flavor)
- ¼ cup Raisins 1 tbsp. Cinnamon 2 cups Water
- Optional Toppings:
- Apple slices Raisins Cinnamon

Directions:
1. Cut the cord and skinned apple into tiny pieces and add them to a saucepan.
2. Add the water and oats to the saucepan and put it over medium heat.
3. Bring to a boil and cook the oats for about 5 minutes.
4. Turn the heat off, add the soy isolate, raisins and cinnamon, then stir thoroughly until everything is well combined. Serve warm with the optional toppings and enjoy!

Nutrition: 366 Calories 4.2g Fat 28g Protein

Paleo Power Bread

Preparation Time: 31 minutes
Cooking Time: 19 minutes
Servings: 8

Ingredients:
- 1 cup Almonds Seven dates (pitted)
- 1 cup Pumpkin seeds
- 1 cup Sunflower seeds 1 cup Flaxseeds
- ¼ cup Water

Directions:
1. Prep the oven to 257°F and line a bread tin with parchment paper.
2. Add all the ingredients to a food processor and blend into a chunky dough.
3. Alternatively, chop the dates into tiny bits, crush the almonds and add them to a large bowl with the remaining ingredients and knead it into a chunky dough by hand.
4. Add the mixture to the bread tin, spread it out from edge to edge and smooth out the top with a tablespoon.
5. Transfer the bread tin to the oven and bake for 20 minutes.
6. Take the bread out of the oven and allow it to cool down completely.

Nutrition: 379 Calories 30.6g Fat 16g Protein

Buckwheat Protein Bread

Preparation Time: 51 minutes
Cooking Time: 38 minutes
Servings: 6

Ingredients:
- 1 cup Buckwheat flour
- ½ cup Pea protein
- ¼ cup Chia seeds
- ¼ cup Raisins
- 3-inch piece Ginger (minced) 2 cups Water

Directions:
1. Set the oven to 190°C and line a small loaf pan with parchment paper.
2. Add all the ingredients except the raisins to a food processor and blend into a smooth and sticky dough.
3. Add the raisins to the dough in the food processor container and stir to distribute them evenly, using a spatula. Transfer the dough to the bread tin, spread it from edge to edge and smooth out the top with a tablespoon. Transfer the bread tin to the oven and bake for 40 minutes.
4. Take the bread out of the oven and allow it to cool down completely.

Nutrition: 151 Calories 9.9g Protein 4.6g Fiber

BREAKFAST RECIPES

Strawberry Muesli

Preparation Time: 19 minutes
Cooking Time: 0 minute
Serving: 3

Ingredients
- One-quarter cup of buckwheat flakes
- Two-thirds cup of buckwheat puffs
- Three tbsp. coconut flakes
- One-quarter cup Medjool dates
- One-eighth cup of chopped walnuts
- One and a half tbsp. of cocoa nibs
- Two-thirds cup of chopped strawberries
- 3/8 cup plain Greek Yoghurt

Direction
1. Simply mix all the ingredients in a clean bowl, and enjoy the fantastic goodness of this delicacy. However, only add strawberries and yogurt when you are ready to eat.

Nutrition: 118 calories 9g fats 6g protein

Sirtfood Omelet

Preparation Time: 8 minutes
Cooking Time: 7 minutes
Serving: 2

Ingredients
- 2 oz. sliced bacon
- Three medium-sized eggs
- One and a one-quarter oz. sliced red endive
- 2 tbsp. chopped parsley
- One tsp. turmeric
- One tsp. extra virgin olive oil

Direction
1. Heat up a non-stick pan.
2. Cut your bacon into thin strips.
3. Cook your sliced bacon strips at high heat until they get crisp and crunchy. You do not have to add oil to the strips; the natural fat would help cook them.
4. Remove the bacon strips from the pan once they're cooked, and place them on a paper towel to drain the extra fat.
5. Wipe your pan clean and then pour in some oil – enough to cook the three eggs.
6. Beat your eggs thoroughly and add in the turmeric, parsley, and endive.
7. Chop your bacon into fine cubes and then stir the bits into the whisked eggs.
8. Pour in oil into your pan and heat at medium heat.
9. Pour the egg mixture in the hot oil and move the mixture around with a spatula
10. Swirl the mixture carefully around the pan until the omelet is even.
11. Lower the heat on your cooker and allow the omelet to firm up and even out at the edges.
12. Fold your omelet in half, roll it up and serve hot.

Nutrition: 291 calories 10g fats 6g protein

Sirtfood Diet Smoothie

Preparation Time: 4 minutes
Cooking Time: 0 minute
Serving: 1

Ingredients
- 3/8 cup of Greek yogurt
- Six walnut halves
- 10 hulled strawberries
- 7 – 10 kale leaves
- ¾ oz. dark chocolate
- One Medjool date
- ½ tsp. ground turmeric
- One sliver of Thai chili
- 200ml of unsweetened almond milk

Direction
1. Load up all the ingredients into your blender and grind into a smooth pulp.

Nutrition: 107 calories 6g fat 3g protein

Yogurt, Berries, Walnuts and Dark Chocolate

Preparation Time: 11 minutes
Cooking Time: 0 minute
Serving: 4

Ingredients
- One and twenty-five grams of mixed berries
- Two-thirds cup of plain Greek yogurt
- ¼ cup of walnuts
- 10g of dark chocolate (85% pure cocoa)

Direction
1. Get a clean bowl and add in your berries.
2. Pour the plain Greek yogurt over the berries
3. Add in your walnuts and dark chocolate, and food is ready.

Nutrition: 188 calories 9g fat 2g protein

Seasoned Scrambled Eggs

Preparation Time: 6 minutes
Cooking Time: 4 minutes
Serving: 3

Ingredients
- One tsp. extra virgin olive oil
- 20g chopped red onions
- ½ chopped Thai chili
- 3 eggs (medium-sized)
- 50 ml of milk
- One tsp ground turmeric
- 2 tbsp. chopped parsley

Direction
1. Place a dry, non-stick frying pan on your cooker and set to medium heat.
2. Fry your chili and red onions till they get soft without being browned.
3. Scourge eggs in a clean bowl and add in the milk, parsley, and turmeric.
4. Pour the mixture into the hot pan and allow to cook at medium heat
5. Spread egg mixture around in the pan to scramble it and prevent burning.
6. Serve once desired consistency is achieved.

Nutrition: 381 calories 16g fats 8g protein

Asian Shrimp Stir-Fry Along with Buckwheat Noodles

Preparation Time: 13 minutes
Cooking Time: 34 minutes
Serving: 4

Ingredients
- Two teaspoons of deveined tamari sauce
- Seventy-five grams of buckwheat noodles
- One hundred and fifty grams of shelled raw jumbo shrimp
- Two pieces of garlic cloves
- One Thai chili (it should be finely chopped)
- One teaspoon of fresh ginger (finely chopped)
- Two teaspoons of extra virgin olive oil
- Twenty grams of red onions
- Forty-five grams of celery (sliced)
- Seventy-five grams of chopped green beans
- Fifty grams of chopped kale
- Half-a-cup of chicken stock

Direction
1. Get a frying pan (non-stick) and then use a high heat setting to heat it up.
2. Proceed by frying the shrimp by using a single teaspoon of tamari sauce along with a single teaspoon of oil. Fry for four minutes.
3. Have the shrimp transferred to a plate then use a clean paper towel to wipe the pan.
4. In the hot water, cook the noodles for five to eight minutes, and strain.
5. Proceed by frying the red onion, green beans, chili, ginger, garlic, kale and celery by using the leftover oil and tamari. Avoid including the celery leaves in that mixture. By using a medium heat setting, fry the ingredients for three-to-four minutes.
6. Now include the stock to your mixture and allow it to cook till the vegs are done.
7. The celery leaves, shrimp and noodles should now be added to the pan. Boil them. Once you're done, lower the heat then serve.

Nutrition: 491 calories 24g fats 18g protein

Miso and Sesame Glazed Tofu with Ginger and Chili Stir

Preparation Time: 14 minutes
Cooking Time: 29 minutes
Serving: 4

Ingredients
- One tbsp mirin
- Twenty grams of miso paste
- One hundred and fifty grams of tofu
- Forty grams of celery
- Forty grams of red onion
- One hundred and twenty grams of zucchini
- One piece of Thai chili
- Two cloves of garlic
- One teaspoon of fresh ginger (finely chopped)

- Fifty grams of kale
- Two teaspoons of sesame seeds
- Thirty-five grams of buckwheat
- One teaspoon of ground turmeric
- Two teaspoons of extra virgin olive oil
- One teaspoon of tamari sauce

Direction
1. Heat your oven to four hundred degrees.
2. Get a small roasting pan and line it with parchment paper.
3. Combine the mirin and the miso.
4. Slice up your tofu lengthwise, and then make each piece out into a triangular shape.
5. Spread the miso mixture over the tofu and allow the tofu to get steeped in the mixture.
6. Cut up your celery, red onion, and zucchini.
7. Cut up the chili, garlic, and ginger.
8. Allow the kale to gently cook in a steamer for five minutes.
9. Transfer your tofu into the roasting pan and spread the sesame seeds over it. Allow the mixture to roast in the oven for twenty minutes.
10. Rinse your buckwheat, and then sieve. Bring a pan filled with water to boil and add in the turmeric.
11. Cook the buckwheat noodles and strain.
12. Allow the oil to heat in a frying pan and then add the celery, onion, zucchini, chili, garlic, and ginger. Allow the entire mix to fry on high heat for two minutes. Reduce the heat to medium for four minutes until the vegetables are cooked.
13. Add a tablespoon of water if the vegetables get stuck to the pan. Spread in the kale and tamari and allow the mixture to cook for another minute.
14. Serve the cooked tofu with the greens and the buckwheat.

Nutrition: 517 calories 26g fats 21g protein

Turkey Escalope with Sage, Parsley & Capers

Preparation Time: 21 minutes
Cooking Time: 42 minutes
Serving: 5
Ingredients
- One hundred and fifty grams of chopped cauliflower
- Two garlic cloves
- Forty grams of red onions
- Two garlic cloves
- One Thai chili
- One teaspoon of chopped fresh ginger
- Two tablespoons of extra virgin olive oil
- Two teaspoons ground turmeric
- Thirty grams of sun-dried tomatoes
- Ten grams of fresh parsley
- One hundred and fifty grams of turkey steak
- One teaspoon of dried sage juice
- One-quarter lemon
- One tablespoon of capers

Direction
1. Put the raw cauliflower into your food processor.
2. Chop up the cauliflower until a fine consistency is achieved.
3. Fry the ginger, garlic, chili and red onions and ginger in the extra virgin olive oil until they are all reasonably soft.
4. Put in your turmeric and cauliflower at this point, and allow the entire mixture to cook for one minute.
5. Bring the mixture down form your cooker, then add the tomatoes and half of your parsley.
6. Cover your turkey escalope with oil and sage and fry for six minutes, making sure to turn carefully to prevent burning.
7. At this point, proceed by pouring in the lemon juice, parsley, capers, and one tablespoon of water to the pan to create your sauce.

Nutrition: 391 calories 24g fats 13g protein

Buckwheat Pancakes, Mushrooms, Red Onions, and Kale Salad

Preparation time: 33 minutes
Cooking Time: 19 minutes
Serving: 5
Ingredients
- One buckwheat pancake
- 50g button mushrooms

- Fifteen grams of chicken
- 200g Kale
- 20g red onions
- Extra Virgin Olive Oil

Direction
1. Clean and cut the button mushrooms.
2. Clean and cut the kale into thin strips and the red onions into rings. Combine the green cabbage and onion in a bowl, season with a drizzle of olive oil, and possibly a little lemon.
3. Cut the chicken into pieces. In a pan, arrange a drizzle of olive oil and add the chicken pieces.
4. Add the mushrooms and brown them.
5. Place everything in the buckwheat pancake, and close the pancake.
6. On a plate, arrange the green cabbage / red onion salad, then place the hot buckwheat pancake next to it. Enjoy your meal!

Nutrition: 387 calories 16g fats 7g protein

Naan Bread with Baked Tofu and Cauliflower

Preparation Time: 17 minutes
Cooking Time: 28 minutes
Serving: 3

Ingredients
- 50 g firm plain tofu
- 50 g cauliflower
- ½ clove garlic
- ½ small onion
- 50ml of water
- 50ml coconut milk
- ½ tablespoon of tomato puree
- ½ teaspoon powdered Indian broth
- ½ tablespoon coconut oil
- ½ teaspoon curry powder
- ½ teaspoon cumin
- ½ tablespoon potato starch

Naan bread:
- 75g wheat flour
- One plain yogurt
- Two pinches of sugar
- 5g baker's yeast or 8 g dehydrated yeast
- 5g salt
- Two tablespoons extra virgin olive oil
- 5 cl lukewarm water
- One teaspoon caraway seed

Direction
1. Peel and mince the garlic and the onions.
2. In a casserole dish, sauté everything in coconut oil with the curry and cumin until lightly colored.
3. Add the coconut milk, the tomato puree, and 50 ml of water and the Indian broth. Mix well then bring to a dainty simmer.
4. Add the tofu pieces and the cauliflower.
5. Cook gently without the lid on for about 20 min until the cauliflower is slightly tender.
6. Dilute the starch with a little cooking juice, then pour back into the casserole dish and continue cooking for 5 min.
7. Serve with basmati rice and naan bread.
8. Naan Bread
9. Put the flour in your food processor.
10. Add the crumbled yeast, olive oil, sugar, yogurt, caraway seeds, and mix well.
11. Proceed by adding the water and continue mixing with the whisk
12. Now place the ball of dough in a small bowl then cover, and allow to stand for thirty minutes.
13. Heat up an empty pan, and cook the naan bread on each side for four minutes to remove moisture.
14. Enjoy your mouth-watering delicacy.

Nutrition: 399 calories 24g fats 16g protein

Sautéed Potatoes in Chicken Broth

Preparation Time: 19 minutes
Cooking Time: 37 minutes
Serving: 6

Ingredients
- Six medium-sized potatoes
- One onion
- Chicken broth
- 100ml of water
- One tbsp extra virgin olive oil
- Salt to taste

Direction
1. First peel the potatoes then slice it across into pieces.
2. Proceed by peeling the onions and chop into small pieces.

3. Fry minced onion pieces in oil for five minutes. Cook the potatoes for 10 minutes while stirring gently.
4. Dilute the chicken broth with water and add to the cooker, and cook for five minutes.
5. Add salt to taste and serve.

Classic Waldorf Salad
Preparation Time: 14 minutes
Cooking Time: 0 minute
Serving: 2
Ingredients
- One hundred and twenty-five grams of mayonnaise
- Two tablespoons white vinegar
- One apple, peeled and cut into pieces
- One celery stalk, diced
- One hundred and twenty-five grams of grapes
- One hundred and twenty-five grams of chopped walnuts
- Salt and pepper to taste

Direction
1. In a large bowl, whisk the mayonnaise and vinegar.
2. Add the apple, celery, raisins, and walnuts.
3. Sprinkle in salt and pepper. Mix everything and serve fresh.

Nutrition: 247 calories 18g fats 11g protein

Whole Wheat Pita
Preparation Time: 1 hour
Cooking Time: 24 minutes
Serving: 8
Ingredients
- 250g of whole wheat flour
- 2 tbsp extra virgin olive oil
- 5g salt
- 10g dry baker's yeast
- One hundred and fifty-ml hot water

Direction
1. Add the whole flour and the salt in a bowl and stir. Then add the rest of the ingredients: oil, yeast, and water. Stir thoroughly to mix.
2. Mix all the ingredients well until the pita bread dough is formed. Knead the dough for a few minutes on the table.
3. Once kneaded, make the dough into a ball and put it in a bowl. Cover and let it be there for two hours.
4. Take out the whole pita bread dough and knead again. Work the dough into balls of about 80g each. Use a roller to make the dough well-rounded. Make the pieces of bread ten-to-twelve cm wide and One cm thick.
5. Put the pitas on a tray. Preheat the oven to 200 ° C, slot in the tray, and let the pieces of bread bake for ten minutes, depending on the oven.
6. Finally, take out the pieces of bread, let them cool a little and serve!

Nutrition: 322 calories 21g fats 16g protein

Scrambled Tofu with Mushrooms
Preparation Time: 8 minutes
Cooking Time: 3 minutes
Serving: 4
Ingredients
- One hundred and twenty-five grams of plain firm tofu
- 100g silky tofu
- One tbsp. fresh cream
- One tbsp. sesame puree
- One tsp. Mustard
- ½ tsp. ground turmeric
- Four sprigs of fresh chives
- Half onion (optional)
- One garlic clove (optional)
- 50g mushrooms
- 2 tbsp. Extra Virgin Olive Oil
- One tbsp. Tamari soy sauce (gluten-free, organic soy sauce)
- Salt and pepper to taste

Direction
1. In a bowl, crush the firm tofu, add in the silky tofu, cream, tahini, mustard, turmeric, and chopped chives.
2. Mix thoroughly, and add salt and pepper to taste.
3. Peel and chop the onion and the garlic.
4. Rinse the mushrooms under a stream of water. Cut off the ends of the stalks and cut the mushrooms into strips. Gently fry the mushrooms, onions, and garlic over

medium-high heat in a pan with a little olive oil.
5. Once the mushrooms, onions, and garlic are very tender and slightly brown in color, add the mixture to the tofu and cook over medium heat for about 5 minutes. Stir the mixture continuously with a spatula.
6. Serve hot, and enjoy.

Nutrition: 276 calories 18g fats 10g protein

Pasta with Smoked Salmon and Arugula

Preparation Time: 13 minutes
Cooking Time: 24 minutes
Serving: 2

Ingredients
- 250g Spaghetti
- One hundred and fifty grams of Smoked salmon
- One bunch of arugulas
- 2 tbsp. Extra virgin olive oil
- One finely chopped onion
- Salt and pepper to taste

Direction
1. Place the pasta in boiling water for ten minutes. Add salt to taste.
2. Slice the smoked salmon into strips. Rinse and wring the arugula.
3. Heat One tablespoonful of extra virgin olive oil in a frying pan and chop the onion. Add in the drained spaghetti, the salmon strips, and the arugula. Mix well and cook for 2 min.
4. Sprinkle in the rest of the olive oil, salt, and pepper.
5. Mix and serve hot.

Nutrition: 477 calories 25g fats 17g protein

Tofu with Cauliflower

Preparation time: 6 minutes
Cooking Time: 45 minutes
Servings 2

Ingredients
- 2 ounces of red pepper, seeded
- 1 Thai chili, cut in two halves, seeded
- 2 cloves of garlic
- 1 teaspoon of olive oil
- 1 pinch of cumin
- 1 pinch of coriander
- Juice of a 1/4 lemon
- 7 ounces of tofu
- 7 ounces of cauliflower, roughly chopped
- 1 ounce of red onions, finely chopped
- 1 teaspoon finely chopped ginger
- 2 teaspoons turmeric
- 2-ounce dried tomatoes, finely chopped
- 2 ounces of parsley, chopped

Direction
1. Preheat oven to 400 °. Slice the peppers and put them in an ovenproof dish with chili and garlic. Pour some olive oil over it, add the dried herbs and put it in the oven for 20 minutes. Let it cool down, put the peppers together with the lemon juice in a blender and work it into a soft mass.
2. Cut the tofu in half and divide the halves into triangles. Place the tofu in a small casserole dish, cover with the paprika mixture and place in the oven for about 20 minutes.
3. Chop the cauliflower until the pieces are smaller than a grain of rice.
4. Then, in a small saucepan, heat the garlic, onions, chili and ginger with olive oil until they become transparent. Add turmeric and cauliflower, mix well and heat again. Remove from heat and add parsley and tomatoes, mix well. Serve with the tofu in the sauce.

Nutrition: 298 Calories 18g fats 11g protein

Indulgent Yoghurt

Preparation Time: 13 minutes
Cooking Time: 24 minutes
Servings: 1

Ingredients
- 125 mixed berries
- 3.5oz of Greek yoghurt
- 25 walnuts, chopped
- 0.9oz of dark chocolate (at least 85% cocoa solids), grated

Directions
1. Toss the mixed berries into a serving bowl. Cover with yoghurt and top with chocolate and walnuts. Voila!

Nutrition: 298 Calories 11g fats 7g protein

Frozen Gazpacho

Preparation Time: 16 minutes
Cooking Time: 0 minutes

Servings: 2
Ingredients:
- 2 large or 6 small tomatoes, chopped
- 1 avocado, seeded, sliced and picked (wait until prompted)
- 1 medium cucumber, chopped
- 1 small red onion, chopped
- 1 cup very finely chopped arugula
- ½ celery stalk, finely chopped
- 1 garlic clove, chopped or pressed
- ½ chili or a pinch of cayenne pepper
- 1 teaspoon of lime juice pinch of sea salt
- A pinch of pepper

Direction:
1. Put the ingredients in a blender or food processor and let them beat gently. You don't want to mix too well, or you make a liquid instead of a soup. The gazpacho must be thick. After mixing, put in the refrigerator for about 1 hour. You can also leave it overnight.
2. Cut and remove the avocado just before eating. Serve half of the gazpacho in a cold bowl. Add the avocado slices and serve immediately.

Nutrition: 292 Calories 13g fat 8g protein

Tomato Frittata

Preparation Time: 17 minutes
Cooking Time: 22 minutes
Servings: 2
Ingredient
- 1.3oz cheddar cheese, grated
- 1.4oz kalamata olives, pitted and halved
- 8 cherry tomatoes, halved
- 4 large eggs
- 1 tablespoon fresh parsley, chopped
- 1 tablespoon fresh basil, chopped
- 1 tablespoon olive oil

Directions
1. Scourge eggs together in a large mixing bowl. Toss in the parsley, basil, olives, tomatoes and cheese, stirring thoroughly.
2. Using small skillet, cook olive oil over high heat. Fill in the frittata mixture and cook for 5-10 minutes. Pull out skillet from the hob and place under the grill for 5 minutes. Divide into portions and serve immediately.

Nutrition: 123 Calories 17g fat 6g protein

Chicken with Kale and Chili Salsa

Preparation Time: 7 minutes
Cooking Time: 41 Minutes
Servings 1
Ingredients
- 3 ounces of buckwheat
- 1 teaspoon of chopped fresh ginger
- Juice of ½ lemon, divided
- 2 teaspoons of ground turmeric
- 3 ounces of kale, chopped
  - ounce of red onion, sliced
- 4 ounce of skinless, boneless chicken breast
- 1 tablespoon of extra-virgin olive oil
- 1 tomato
- 1 handful parsley
- 1 bird's eye chili, chopped

Directions
1. Start with the salsa: Remove the eye out of the tomato and finely chop it. Mix it with the chili, parsley, and lemon juice.
2. Heat your oven to 220 degrees F. Marinate the chicken with a little oil, 1 teaspoon of turmeric, and the lemon juice. Let it rest for 5-10 minutes.
3. Preheat pan over medium heat until it is hot then add marinated chicken and allow it to cook for a minute on both sides until it is pale gold. Transfer the chicken to the oven and bake for 10 minutes. Get the chicken out of the oven, cover with foil, and rest for five minutes before you serve.
4. Meanwhile, in a steamer, steam the kale for about 5 minutes.
5. In a little oil, fry the ginger and red onions until they are soft but not colored, and then add in the cooked kale and fry it for a minute.
6. Cook the buckwheat in accordance to the packet Directions with the remaining turmeric. Serve alongside the vegetables, salsa and chicken.

Nutrition: 135 Calories 15g fats 9g protein

Buckwheat Tuna Casserole

Preparation Time: 9 minutes
Cooking Time: 38 minutes

Servings: 2

Ingredients

- 2 tablespoons butter
- 10-ounce package buckwheat ramen noodles
- 2 cups boiling water
- 1/3 cup dry red wine
- 3 cups milk
- 2 tablespoons dried parsley
- 2 teaspoons turmeric
- ½ teaspoon curry powder
- 2 tablespoons All-Purpose flour
- 2 cups celery, chopped
- 1 cup frozen peas
- 2 cans tuna, drained

Directions

1. Dot butter into your crockpot and grease the pot.
2. Place buckwheat ramen noodles in a large bowl and pour boiling water to cover. Let sit for 5 – 8 minutes, or until noodles separate when prodded with a fork.
3. Scourge red wine, milk, parsley, turmeric and flour.
4. Fold in celery, peas, and tuna.
5. Drain the ramen and place into crockpot, pouring the tuna mixture over top. Mix to combine.
6. Close and cook at Low 8 hours, stirring occasionally.

Nutrition: 411 Calories 19g fats 11g protein

Tuscan Stewed Beans

Preparation Time: 21 minutes
Cooking Time: 33 minutes
Servings: 1

Ingredients

- 1 dl. extra virgin olive oil
- Salt to taste
- Pepper as needed.
- Cannellini beans
- Sage
- Garlic clove
- Water

Directions

1. Submerge beans for at least 12 hours before cooking. Pour the beans in a crockpot with water, a clove of garlic, sage, and a generous pinch of salt, adjust the flame as low as possible.
2. Once boiling, cover the pot, and continue cooking for at least 3 and a half hours, taking care that the flame remains very low, the beans in the pot must not move around.
3. Once you are done cooking, serve the beans with extra virgin olive oil, salt, and pepper on the table.

Nutrition: 145 Calories 22g fats 15g protein

Buckwheat Tabbouleh with Strawberries

Preparation Time: 21 minutes
Cooking Time: 33 minutes
Servings: 1

Ingredients

- Buckwheat (broken)
- Turmeric powder 2 teaspoon
- Avocado 1
- Tomatoes
- Tropia red onions
- Medjool dates (pitted)
- Parsley
- Strawberries
- 2 tablespoons extra virgin olive oil
- Lemon juice 1
- Rocket 1.3 ounce

Direction

1. Heat up the water to cook the buckwheat.
2. When it boils, add turmeric and buckwheat. Be careful not to overcook it. It is good to leave, it "al dente." When cooked, drain the buckwheat and set aside to cool. Take a large bowl to spice the tabbouleh.
3. Cut the tomatoes into cubes and let them drain for a few minutes in a colander to remove the water.
4. On a cutting board, begin to finely chop the red onion, dates, and parsley and combine them with buckwheat.
5. Skin the avocado and cut it into small cubes and add it with the tomatoes to the buckwheat. Cut the strawberries into slices and gently add them to the rest of the ingredients. Add the chopped arugula, oil, and lemon juice. Mix all the ingredients

and let the buckwheat tabbouleh take on extra flavor for an hour before serving it at the table.

Nutrition: 145 Calories 26g fat 13g protein

Scramble Tofu and Mushroom

Preparation Time: 11 minutes
Cooking Time: 28 minutes
Servings: 2

Ingredients
- 7 ounces of extra firm tofu
- 2 teaspoon turmeric powder
- 1 teaspoon black pepper
- ounce of kale, roughly chopped
- 2 teaspoons extra virgin olive oil
- Oz. of red onion
- 1 Thai chili
- 100g mushrooms
- 4 tbsp. parsley

Direction
1. Drain tofu in paper towels.
2. Blend the turmeric with water.
3. Steam the kale for 3 minutes.
4. Cook olive oil at medium heat, fry onion, chili, and mushrooms for 3 minutes
5. Crush the tofu into bite-size pieces and put in the pan, mix the turmeric paste over the tofu. Season with black pepper. Cook at medium heat for 2 minutes
6. Cook kale at medium heat for 4 minutes. Sprinkle parsley and serve.

Nutrition: 122 calories 20g fat 11g protein

Kale Scramble

Preparation Time: 17 minutes
Cooking Time: 6 minutes
Servings: 2

Ingredients
- 4 eggs
- 1/8 teaspoon ground turmeric
- Salt and ground black pepper, to taste
- 1 tablespoon water
- 2 teaspoons olive oil
- 1 cup fresh kale, tough ribs removed and chopped

Directions
1. Scourge eggs, turmeric, salt, black pepper, and water and using a whisk.
2. In a wok, cook oil over medium heat.
3. Stir egg mixture and stir to combine.
4. Set the heat to medium-low and cook for 2 minutes.
5. Mix in the kale and cook for 4 minutes.
6. Remove from the heat and serve immediately.

Nutrition: 183 Calories 25g fats 13g protein

Pancakes with Blackcurrant Compote

Preparation Time: 18 minutes
Cooking Time: 21 minutes
Servings: 2

Ingredients
- 4 ounce of porridge oats
- ounce of plain flour
- 1 tablespoon caster sugar
- ½ teaspoon baking powder
- 1 large green apple
- 2/3 cup semi-skimmed milk
- 1 egg white
- 1 tsp. olive oil.

For the compote:
- ounce of blackcurrants washed and stalks removed.
- 1 tablespoon caster sugar
- 2 tablespoon water.

Direction
For compote:
1. Simmer blackcurrants, sugar, and water for 13 minutes.

For Pancake:
2. Incorporate Oats, flour, baking powder, and caster sugar in a bowl.
3. Mix apple into the powder mixture then stir in milk simultaneously.
4. Beat egg white to a stiff peak then mix into the pancake batter.
5. Pre-heat ½ teaspoon olive oil in a non-stick frying pan at medium heat and place ½ of the batter. Lower the heat then cook both sides until golden brown.
6. Drizzle pancakes with the blackcurrant compote.

Nutrition: 123 calories 20g fats 8g protein

Cinnamon Buckwheat Porridge

Preparation Time: 12 minutes

Cooking Time: 17 minutes
Servings: 2
Ingredients
- 1 cup buckwheat, rinsed
- 1 cup unsweetened almond milk
- 1 cup water
- ½ teaspoon ground cinnamon
- ½ teaspoon vanilla extract
- 1–2 tablespoons raw honey
- ¼ cup fresh blueberries

Directions
1. Boil all the ingredients (except honey and blueberries) at medium-high heat
2. Now, reduce the heat to low and simmer, covered for about 10 minutes.
3. Drizzle honey and take out from the heat.
4. Set aside, covered, for 5 minutes.
5. With a fork, fluff the mixture, and transfer into serving bowls.
6. Top with blueberries and serve.

Nutrition: 358 Calories 29g fats 18g protein

Mushroom Scramble Egg

Preparation Time: 7 minutes
Cooking Time: 13 minutes
Servings: 3
Ingredients
- Two eggs
- 1 teaspoon ground turmeric
- 1 teaspoon mild curry powder
- 20g kale, roughly chopped
- 1 teaspoon extra virgin olive oil
- ½ bird's eye chili, thinly sliced
- A handful of thinly sliced, button mushrooms
- 5g parsley, finely chopped

Directions
1. Mix the curry and turmeric powder, then add a little water until a light paste has been achieved.
2. Steam up the kale 2–3 minutes.
3. Over medium heat, cook oil in a frying pan and fry the chili and mushrooms for 2–3 minutes
4. Put the eggs and spice paste, and cook over medium heat, then add the kale and start cooking for another minute over medium heat. Add the parsley, then mix well and serve.

Nutrition: 185 Calories 27g fats 16g protein

Sirtfood Eggs and Mushroom

Preparation Time: 13 minutes
Cooking Time: 21 minutes
Servings: 1
Ingredients
- 2 medium eggs
- 1 teaspoon turmeric
- 1 ounce of kale, roughly chopped
- 1 teaspoon extra virgin olive oil
- 1/2 chili, thinly sliced
- 0.5 ounce of red onions
- Parsley, thinly chopped
- A handful of button mushrooms, thinly sliced

Direction
1. Smoke the kale for 2 minutes.
2. Dissolve turmeric powder with water.
3. Blend turmeric paste, parsley, and mix properly.
4. Warm up olive oil at medium heat then sauté onion, chili, and mushroom
5. Mix steamed kale to the mix in the frying pan.
6. Stir in egg mixture to the pan
7. Decrease heat and cook the egg.

Nutrition: 157 Calories 52g Protein 26g fats

Matcha Green Juice

Preparation Time: 8 minutes
Cooking time: 0 minutes
Servings: 2
Ingredients
- 5 ounces fresh kale
- 2 ounces fresh arugula
- ¼ cup fresh parsley
- ½ tsp. Matcha green tea
- 4 celery stalks
- 1 green apple, cored and chopped
- 1 (1-inch) piece fresh ginger, peeled
- 1 lemon, peeled

Direction
1. Incorporate the all ingredients then extract the juice as stated by the manufacturer's direction.
2. Fill into the glasses then serve.

Nutrition: 115 Calories 27g fat 11g protein

Berry Pancakes

Preparation Time: 11 minutes
Cooking Time: 4 minutes
Servings: 4

Ingredients
- ½ cup coconut milk
- 1 tablespoon coconut oil
- 1 egg, beaten lightly
- 1/3 cup buckwheat flour
- 1 teaspoon baking powder
- Pinch of salt
- ¼ cup frozen blueberries

Direction
1. Incorporate flour, baking powder, and salt.
2. Scourge coconut milk, coconut oil, and eggs.
3. Stir in flour mixture and mix well.
4. Fold in blueberries.
5. Heat up greased non-stick skillet at medium heat.
6. Place half of the mixture and spread in an even circle.
7. Cook for about 2–3 minutes.
8. Flip and cook for additional 1 minute.
9. Repeat with the remaining mixture.
10. Serve warm.

Nutrition: 181 Calories 11g Fat 5.4g Protein

Pumpkin Pancakes

Preparation Time: 13 minutes
Cooking Time: 41 minutes
Servings: 10

Ingredients
- 2 tablespoons ground flaxseed
- 6 tablespoons water
- 1 cup buckwheat flour
- 1 tablespoon baking powder
- 1 teaspoon pumpkin pie spice
- ½ teaspoon salt
- 1 cup pumpkin puree
- ¾ cup plus 2 tablespoons unsweetened almond milk
- 3 tablespoons pure maple syrup
- 2 tablespoons coconut oil
- 1 teaspoon vanilla extract

Direction:
1. Mix ground flaxseed well. Set aside for 5 minutes.
2. In a blender, add flaxseed mixture and remaining ingredients and pulse until well combined.
3. Situate mixture into a bowl and set aside for about 10 minutes.
4. Preheat greased non-stick skillet over medium heat.
5. Place about ¼ cup of the mixture and spread in an even circle.
6. Cook for about 2 minutes per side.
7. Repeat with the remaining mixture.
8. Serve warm.

Nutrition: 102 Calories 4g Fat 2.1g Protein

Simple Waffles

Preparation Time: 12 minutes
Cooking Time: 40 minutes
Servings: 4

Ingredients
- 1¼ cups unsweetened almond milk
- 1 tablespoon apple cider vinegar
- 1 tablespoon ground flaxseed
- 3 tablespoons water
- 1 cup buckwheat flour
- 1 tablespoon coconut sugar
- 1¼ teaspoons baking powder
- 1 teaspoon baking soda
- ¼ teaspoon salt
- ¼ teaspoon ground cinnamon

Direction
1. In a cup, mix together almond milk vinegar. Set aside for 5 minutes.
2. Incorporate ground flaxseed. Keep aside for 6 minutes.
3. In a separate bowl, add buckwheat flour, coconut sugar, cinnamon, baking powder, baking soda, and salt, and mix well.
4. In the bowl of flaxseed mixture, add almond milk mixture and stir to combine.
5. Mix flour mixture. Set aside for about 8 minutes.
6. Heat and grease the waffle iron
7. Place the desired amount of the mixture into the preheated waffle iron and cook for about 5 minutes per side or until golden-brown.
8. Repeat with the remaining mixture.
9. Serve warm.

Nutrition: 136 Calories 2.6g Fat 4.4g Protein

Green Veggies Quiche

Preparation Time: 17 minutes
Cooking Time: 17 minutes
Servings: 4

Ingredients

- 6 eggs
- ½ cup unsweetened almond milk
- Salt and ground black pepper, to taste
- 2 cups fresh baby kale, chopped
- ½ cup green bell pepper, seeded and chopped
- 1 scallion, chopped
- ¼ cup fresh parsley, chopped
- 1 tablespoon fresh chives, minced

Direction

1. Preheat the oven to 400°F.
2. Lightly grease a pie dish.
3. In a bowl, add eggs, almond milk, salt, and black pepper, and beat until well combined. Set aside.
4. In another bowl, add the vegetables and herbs and mix well.
5. In the bottom of prepared pie dish, place the veggie mixture evenly and top with the egg mixture.
6. Bake for 21 minutes.
7. Remove pie dish from the oven and set aside for about 5 minutes before slicing.
8. Cut into desired sized wedges and serve warm.

Nutrition: 123 Calories 7.1g Fat 9.8g Protein

Tofu & Kale Omelet

Preparation Time: 21 minutes
Cooking Time: 23 minutes
Servings: 2

Ingredients

- 10 ounces firm silken tofu, pressed and drained
- 4 tablespoons nutritional yeast
- 4 tablespoons hummus
- 2 teaspoons arrowroot powder
- 2 cups fresh kale, tough ribs removed and chopped
- ½ teaspoon paprika
- Salt and ground black pepper, to taste
- 1–2 tablespoons water
- 2 tablespoons extra-virgin olive oil

Direction

1. Preheat oven to 375°F.
2. Using a food processor, blend tofu, nutritional yeast, hummus, arrowroot powder, paprika, salt, black pepper, and water.
3. Grease a medium, ovenproof skillet with 1 tablespoon of oil and heat over medium heat.
4. Add the kale, salt, and black pepper, and sauté for about 3–5 minutes.
5. Remove from the heat and transfer the kale into a bowl.
6. Grease the same skillet with the remaining oil.
7. In the bottom of greases skillet, place the tofu mixture.
8. With a spatula, gently spread the tofu mixture in a thin and even layer.
9. Situate skillet over medium heat and cook for 5 minutes.
10. Immediately, transfer the skillet into the oven and bake for about 10–15 minutes
11. In the last 5 minutes of cooking, situate remaining cooked kale on top evenly.
12. Remove the skillet from oven and fold over the omelet.
13. Cut the omelet in 2 portions and serve.

Nutrition: 371 Calories 21.7g Fat 23.3g Protein

Kale, Chickpeas & Olives Salad

Preparation Time: 18 minutes
Cooking Time: 0 minutes
Servings: 4

Ingredients

Dressing

- 2 tablespoons fresh orange juice
- 2 tablespoons fresh lemon juice
- 3 tablespoons extra-virgin olive oil
- 1 tablespoon red wine vinegar
- 1 tablespoon honey
- 1 tablespoon fresh orange zest, grated
- ¾ tablespoon Dijon mustard
- Salt and ground black pepper, to taste

Salad

- 3 cups cooked chickpeas
- 2 cups mixed olives, pitted
- 1 cup red onion, chopped

- 6 cups fresh kale, tough ribs removed and torn

Direction
1. For dressing: In a small bowl, add all ingredients and beat well.
2. For salad: In a large salad bowl, mix together all ingredients.
3. Place dressing over salad and toss to coat well.
4. Serve immediately.

Nutrition: 468 Calories 20g Fat 13.1g Protein

Steak Salad

Preparation Time: 21 minutes
Cooking Time: 7 minutes
Servings: 2

Ingredients
Steak
- 1 (12-ounce) sirloin steak
- Salt and ground black pepper, to taste
- 2 tablespoons extra-virgin olive oil

Salad
- ¼ cup cucumber; peeled, seeded, and sliced
- ¼ cup red onion, sliced
- ¼ cup cherry tomatoes, halved
- 2 tablespoons fresh parsley, chopped
- 2 tablespoons fresh mint leaves
- 3 cups fresh kale, tough ribs removed and chopped finely

Dressing
- 1 tablespoon extra-virgin olive oil
- 1 tablespoon fresh lemon juice
- Salt and ground black pepper, to taste

Direction
1. For steak: Season the steak with salt and black pepper lightly.
2. In a heavy-bottomed sauté pan, heat 2 tablespoons of the oil over high heat and cook the steak for 8 minutes on both sides.
3. Pull out from the heat and place the steak onto a cutting board for about 10 minutes.
4. For salad: Place all ingredients in a salad bowl and mix.
5. For dressing: Place all ingredients in another bowl and beat until well combined.
6. Cut the steaks into desired sized slices against the grain.
7. Place the salad onto each serving plate.
8. Top each plate with steak slices.
9. Drizzle with dressing and serve.

Nutrition: 567 Calories 31.8g Fat 55g Protein

Chicken & Orange Salad

Preparation Time: 13 minutes
Cooking Time: 16 minutes
Servings: 5

Ingredients
Chicken
- 4 (6-ounce) boneless, skinless chicken breast halves
- Salt and ground black pepper, to taste
- 2 tablespoons extra-virgin olive oil

Salad
- 8 cups fresh baby arugula
- 5 medium oranges, peeled and sectioned
- 1 cup onion, sliced

Dressing
- 2 tablespoons extra-virgin olive oil
- 2 tablespoons fresh orange juice
- 2 tablespoons red wine vinegar
- 1½ teaspoons shallots, minced
- 1 garlic clove, minced
- Salt and ground black pepper, to taste

Direction
1. For chicken: Season each chicken breast half with salt and black pepper evenly.
2. Place chicken over a rack set in a rimmed baking sheet.
3. Refrigerate for at least 30 minutes.
4. Remove the baking sheet from refrigerator and pat dry the chicken breast halves with paper towels.
5. Heat the oil in a 12-inch sauté pan over medium-low heat.
6. Place the chicken breast halves, smooth-side down, and cook for about 9–10 minutes, without moving.
7. Flip the chicken breasts and cook for about 6 minutes or until cooked through.
8. Remove the sauté pan from heat and let the chicken stand in the pan for about 3 minutes.
9. Transfer the chicken breasts onto a cutting board for about 5 minutes.
10. Cut each chicken breast half into desired-sized slices.

11. For salad: Place all ingredients in a salad bowl and mix.
12. Add chicken slices and stir to combine.
13. For dressing: place all ingredients in another bowl and beat until well combined.
14. Place the salad onto each serving plate.
15. Drizzle with dressing and serve.

Nutrition: 463 Calories 22g Fat 42g Protein

Buckwheat Burgers

Preparation Time: 18 minutes
Cooking Time: 47 minutes
Servings: 4

Ingredients

Patties
- ¾ cup dry buckwheat
- 1½ cups filtered water
- Salt, to taste
- 2 tablespoons extra-virgin olive oil, divided
- ½ of large yellow onion, chopped finely
- ½ of large carrot, peeled and grated
- ½ of celery stalk, chopped finely
- 1 fresh kale leaf, tough ribs removed and chopped finely
- 1 cooked sweet potato
- 2 tablespoons almond butter
- 2 tablespoons low-sodium soy sauce

Salad
- 4 cups fresh baby arugula
- 2 large tomatoes, chopped

Direction
1. Preheat the oven to 350°F.
2. Line a baking sheet with parchment paper.
3. For patties: Heat a non-stick frying pan over medium heat and toast the buckwheat for about 5 minutes, stirring continuously.
4. Boil water and salt over high heat.
5. Put heat to low and cook, covered for 15 minutes.
6. Cook 1 tablespoon of the oil in a skillet over medium heat and sauté the onion for 5 minutes.
7. Cook carrot and celery for 5 minutes.
8. Stir in the remaining ingredients and remove from the heat.
9. Transfer the mixture into a bowl with buckwheat and stir to combine.
10. Set aside to cool completely.
11. Make 4 equal-sized patties from the mixture.
12. Arrange the patties onto the prepared baking sheet in a single layer and bake for about
13. Bake for about 20 minutes per side.
14. Divide the arugula and tomatoes onto serving plates.
15. Top each plate with 2 patties and serve

Nutrition: 287 Calories 21.7g Fat 8.3g Protein

Sautéed Mushrooms

Preparation Time: 16 minutes
Cooking Time: 11 minutes
Servings: 2

Ingredients
- 2 tablespoons extra-virgin olive oil
- 2–3 tablespoons red onion, minced
- ½ teaspoon garlic, minced
- 12 ounces fresh mushrooms, sliced
- 1 tablespoon fresh parsley
- 1 teaspoon fresh lemon juice
- Salt and ground black pepper, to taste

Direction
1. In a sauté pan, heat the oil over medium heat and sauté the onion and garlic for 3–4 minutes.
2. Cook mushrooms and cook for 9 minutes.
3. Stir in the parsley, lemon juice, salt and black pepper and remove from the heat.
4. Serve hot.

Nutrition: 163 Calories 14.5g Fat 5.6g Protein

Kale with Cranberries & Pine Nuts

Preparation Time: 13 minutes
Cooking Time: 17 minutes
Servings: 6

Ingredients
- 2 pounds fresh kale, tough ribs removed and chopped
- 3 tablespoons extra-virgin olive oil
- 1 tablespoon garlic, minced
- ½ cup dried unsweetened cranberries
- Salt and ground black pepper, to taste
- 1/3 cup pine nuts

Direction
1. Using a pan of boiling salted water, cook the kale for about 5–7 minutes.

2. In a colander, drain the kale and immediately transfer into an ice bath.
3. Drain the kale and set aside.
4. Preheat oil on medium heat and sauté the garlic for about 1 minute.
5. Add kale, cranberries, salt, and black pepper, and cook for about 4–6 minutes, tossing frequently with tongs.
6. Stir in the pine nuts and serve hot.

Nutrition: 196 Calories 12.2g Fat 5.6g Protein

Tofu with Kale

Preparation Time: 18 minutes
Cooking Time: 8 minutes
Servings: 2

Ingredients
- 1 tablespoon extra-virgin olive oil
- ½ pound tofu; pressed, drained, and cubed
- 1 teaspoon fresh ginger, minced
- 1 garlic clove, minced
- ¼ teaspoon red pepper flakes, crushed
- 6 ounces fresh kale, tough ribs removed and chopped finely
- 1 tablespoon low-sodium soy sauce

Direction
1. Pre-heat olive oil in a large non-stick wok over medium-high heat and stir-fry the tofu for about 2–3 minutes.
2. Sauté ginger, garlic and red pepper flakes, stirring continuously.
3. Stir in the kale and soy sauce and stir-fry for about 4–5 minutes.
4. Serve hot.

Nutrition: 190 Calories 11.8g Fat 12.5g Protein

Buckwheat Pancakes

Preparation Time: 11 minutes
Cooking Time: 17 minutes
Servings: 5

Ingredients
- 1 cup unsweetened almond milk
- 2 teaspoons apple cider vinegar
- 1 cup buckwheat flour
- 2 tablespoons ground flaxseed
- 1 tablespoon baking powder
- ¼ teaspoon sea salt
- ¼ cup maple syrup
- 1 teaspoon vanilla extract
- 1 tablespoon extra-virgin olive oil

Direction
1. Blend almond milk and vinegar. Set aside.
2. Combine flour, flaxseed, baking powder, and salt.
3. Add the coconut milk mixture, maple syrup, and vanilla extract and beat until well combined.
4. In a non-stick skillet, heat the oil over medium heat.
5. Transfer 1/3 cup of the mix in a pan and spread in an even circle.
6. Cook for about 1–2 minutes.
7. Flip and cook for additional 1 minute.
8. Repeat with the remaining mixture.
9. Serve warm.

Nutrition: 174 Calories 5.2g Fat 3.8g Protein

Blueberry Waffles

Preparation Time: 14 minutes
Cooking Time: 21 minutes
Servings: 2

Ingredients
- ¼ cup coconut flour
- ½ teaspoon baking powder
- Pinch of salt
- 1/8 teaspoon ground cinnamon
- 4 eggs
- ¼ cup coconut oil, melted
- 2 tablespoons maple syrup
- 1 tablespoon fresh lemon juice
- ¼ cup fresh blueberries
- 1½ teaspoons lemon zest, grated

Direction
1. Through a fine-mesh sieve, sift together the flour, baking powder, cinnamon, and salt in a bowl.
2. In another large bowl, add the eggs and coconut oil and beat until well combined.
3. Add the maple syrup and lemon juice and again beat until well combined.
4. Stir in flour mixture and combine well.
5. Lightly, stir in blueberries and lemon zest.
6. Heat waffle iron and grease, it.
7. Pour desired amount of mixture and cook for about 5 minutes or until golden-brown.
8. Repeat with the remaining mixture.
9. Serve warm.

Nutrition: 244 Calories 19g Fat 6.7g Protein

Tofu & Arugula Scramble

Preparation Time: 13 minutes

Cooking Time: 9 minutes
Servings: 2

Ingredients

- 1 tablespoon extra-virgin olive oil
- 1 garlic clove, minced
- ¼ pound medium-firm tofu, drained, pressed, and crumbled
- 1/3 cup homemade vegetable broth
- 2½ cups fresh arugula
- ¼ cup tomato, chopped finely
- 2 teaspoons low-sodium soy sauce
- 1 teaspoon ground turmeric
- 1 teaspoon fresh lemon juice

Direction

1. Cook olive oil in a frying pan over medium-high heat and sauté the garlic for about 1 minute.
2. Add the tofu and cook for about 2–3 minutes, slowly adding the broth.
3. Add the arugula, tomato, soy sauce, and turmeric and stir fry for about 3–4 minutes. Drizzle lemon juice and serve immediately.

Nutrition: 125 Calories 10g Fat 6.8g Protein

MAIN DISH RECIPES

Aromatic Chicken Breast, Kale, Red Onion, and Salsa

Preparation Time: 53 minutes
Cooking Time: 32 minutes
Servings: 2

Ingredients

- 120g skinless, boneless chicken breast
- 2 teaspoons ground turmeric
- ¼ lemon
- 1 tablespoon extra-virgin olive oil
- 50g kale, chopped
- 20g red onion, sliced
- 1 teaspoon fresh ginger, chopped
- 50g buckwheat

Directions

1. To prepare the salsa, remove the tomato eye and finely chop. Add the chili, parsley, capers, lemon juice and mix.
2. Set oven to 220°C. Pour 1 teaspoon of the turmeric, the lemon juice and a little oil on the chicken breast and marinate. Allow to stay for 5–10 minutes.
3. Position an ovenproof frying pan on the heat and cook the marinated chicken for a minute on each side to achieve a pale golden color. Then transfer the pan containing the chicken to the oven and allow to stay for 8–10 minutes or until it is done. Pull out from the oven and wrap with foil, set aside for 5 minutes before serving.
4. Situate kale in a steamer for 5 minutes. Drizzle little oil in a frying pan and sauté red onions and the ginger. Stir in cooked kale and fry for another minute.
5. Cook the buckwheat following the packet's instructions using the remaining turmeric. Serve alongside the chicken, salsa, and vegetables.

Nutrition: 149 Calories 16g Protein 5g Fat

Kale and Red Onion Dal with Buckwheat

Preparation Time 7 minutes
Cooking Time 25 minutes
Servings: 2

Ingredients

- ½ tablespoon olive oil
- ½ small red onion, sliced
- 1 ½ garlic cloves, crushed
- 1cm ginger, grated
- ½ birds eye chili, deseeded and finely chopped
- 1 teaspoon turmeric
- 1 teaspoon garam masala
- 80g red lentils
- 200ml coconut milk
- 100ml water
- 50g kale or spinach
- 80g buckwheat or brown rice

Directions

1. Cook olive oil, stir in sliced onion and cook on a low heat for 5 minutes. Sauté ginger, garlic, and chili for extra 1 minute.
2. Add to it, the garam masala, turmeric, and a splash of water. Cook for 3 minutes before adding the coconut milk, red lentils, and 200ml water.
3. Thoroughly mix all together and cook over a gentle heat for 20 minutes with the lid closed. When the dhal starts sticking, add a little more water and stir occasionally.
4. Add the kale, after 20 minutes and thoroughly stir and still cover the lid to cook for additional 5 minutes or 1-2 minutes when you substitute with spinach.
5. Put the buckwheat in a saucepan and pour boiling water like 15 minutes before the curry gets ready. Allow the water to boil and cook for 10-12 minutes. Drain the buckwheat and serve with the dhal.

Nutrition: 355 Calories 14g Protein 5.7g Fat

Chargrilled Beef and Herb Roasted Potatoes

Preparation Time: 90 minutes
Cooking Time: 70 minutes
Servings: 2

Ingredients

- 100g potatoes, peeled and dice
- 1 tablespoon extra-virgin olive oil
- 5g parsley, finely chopped
- 50g red onion, sliced into rings

- 50g kale, sliced
- 1 garlic clove, finely chopped
- 120–150g beef fillet steak
- 40ml red wine
- 150ml beef stock
- 1 teaspoon tomato purée
- 1 teaspoon corn flour
- 1 tablespoon water

Directions
1. Preheat the oven to 220C (430F) and put the potatoes in a boiling water and cook for 4–5 minutes, drain. Pour 1 teaspoon oil in a roasting tin and roast the potatoes for 35–45 minutes turning the potatoes on every sides every 10 minutes to ensure they cook evenly.
2. Remove from the oven when fully cooked, sprinkle with chopped parsley and mix thoroughly.
3. Pour 1 teaspoon of the oil on a saucepan and fry the onion for 5-7 minutes to become soft and neatly caramelized. Keep it warm.
4. Place the kale in a saucepan, steam for 2–3 minutes and drain. In ½ teaspoon of oil, fry the garlic for 1 minute to become soft though not colored. Add the kale and continue to fry for extra 1–2 minutes to become tender. Maintain the warmth.
5. Over a high heat, place an ovenproof frying pan until it becomes smoking. Then use the ½ a teaspoon of the oil to coat the meat and fry over a medium–high heat. Take out the meat and set aside to rest.
6. Pour the wine to the hot pan and bubble to reduce the wine quantity by half to form syrupy and to have a concentrated flavor. Add the tomato purée and stock to the steak pan and boil. Add the corn flour paste little at a time to act as a thickener to until the desired consistency is achieved. Add any juices from the rested steak and serve with the kale, onion rings, roasted potatoes, and red wine sauce.

Nutrition: 244 Calories 14g Protein 14.4g Fat

Crunchy Braised Leeks

Preparation Time: 41 minutes
Cooking Time: 21 minutes
Servings: 3

Ingredients
- 20 g Ghee
- 2 teaspoon Olive oil
- 2 pieces Leek
- 150 ml Vegetable broth
- Fresh parsley
- 1 tablespoon fresh oregano
- 1 tablespoon Pine nuts

Directions
1. Cut the leek into thin rings and finely chop the herbs. Roast the pine nuts in a dry pan over medium heat.
2. Melt the ghee together with the olive oil in a large pan.
3. Cook the leek until golden brown for 5 minutes, stirring constantly.
4. Add the vegetable broth and cook for another 10 minutes.
5. Stir in the herbs and drizzle pine nuts on the dish just before serving.

Nutrition: 95 Calories 1.35g Protein 4.8g Fat

Sweet and Sour Pan with Cashew Nuts

Preparation Time: 31 minutes
Cooking Time: 0 minutes
Servings: 2

Ingredients
- 2 tablespoon Coconut oil
- 2 pieces Red onion
- 2 pieces yellow bell pepper
- 250 g White cabbage
- 150 g Pak choy
- 50 g Mung bean sprouts
- 4 pieces Pineapple slices
- 50 g Cashew nuts
- For the sweet and sour sauce:
- 60 ml Apple cider vinegar
- 4 tablespoon Coconut blossom sugar
- 2 tablespoon Tomato paste
- 1 teaspoon Coconut-Aminos
- 2 teaspoon Arrowroot powder
- 75 ml Water

Directions
1. Roughly cut the vegetables.
2. Mix the arrow root with five tablespoons of cold water into a paste.

3. Situate all the other ingredients for the sauce in a saucepan and add the arrowroot paste for binding.
4. Cook coconut oil in a pan and fry the onion.
5. Add the bell pepper, cabbage, Pak choy and bean sprouts and stir-fry until the vegetables become a little softer.
6. Add the pineapple and cashew nuts and stir a few more times.
7. Pour a little sauce over the wok dish and serve.

Nutrition: 573 Calories 15.2g Protein 27.8g Fat

Eggplant and Spinach Casserole

Preparation Time: 60 minutes
Cooking Time: 42 minutes
Servings: 3

Ingredients
- 1 Eggplant
- 2 Onions
- Olive oil 3 tbsp.
- Spinach 16 oz.
- 4 Tomatoes
- 2 Egg
- ¼ cup Almond milk
- 2 tsp. Lemon juice
- 4 tbsp. Almond flour

Directions
1. Set oven to 200°C
2. Slice eggplants, onions and tomatoes and rub with salt.
3. Fry eggplants and onions with olive oil in a grill pan.
4. Blanch spinach in a saucepan at medium heat and strain.
5. Arrange vegetables in layers in a greased baking dish: eggplant, spinach, onion and tomato in this order. Repeat.
6. Scourge eggs with almond milk, lemon juice, salt and pepper then drizzle over the vegetables.
7. Dust some almond flour and bake for 36 minutes.

Nutrition: 443 Calories 11g Protein 33g Fat

Vegetarian Paleo Ratatouille

Preparation Time: 71 minutes
Cooking Time: 52 minutes
Servings: 2

Ingredients
- 200 g (7 oz.) Tomato cubes (can)
- ½ pieces Onion
- 2 cloves Garlic
- ¼ teaspoon dried oregano
- ¼ TL Chili flakes
- 2 tablespoon Olive oil
- 1-piece Eggplant
- 1-piece Zucchini
- 1-piece hot peppers
- 1 teaspoon dried thyme

Directions
1. Prepare oven to 180°C and slightly grease a round dish.
2. Slice the onion and garlic.
3. Incorporate tomato cubes with garlic, onion, oregano and chili flakes, season well and situate on the bottom of the baking dish.
4. With a mandolin, cut the eggplant, zucchini and hot pepper into very thin slices.
5. Place vegetables in a bowl
6. Pour the remaining olive oil on the vegetables and season with thyme, salt and pepper.
7. Wrap baking dish with parchment paper and bake for 51 minutes.

Nutrition: 273 Calories 5.6g Protein 14.5g Fat

Vegetarian Curry from the Crock Pot

Preparation Time: 6 hours
Cooking Time: 6 hours
Servings: 2

Ingredients
- 4 pieces Carrot
- 2 pieces Sweet potato
- 1-piece Onion
- 3 cloves Garlic
- 2 tablespoon Curry powder
- 1 teaspoon Ground caraway (ground)
- ¼ teaspoon Chili powder
- ¼ TL Celtic sea salt
- 1 pinch Cinnamon
- 100 ml (3 ½ fl. oz.) Vegetable broth
- 400 g (14 oz.) Tomato cubes (can)

- 250 g (9 oz.) Sweet peas
- 2 tablespoon Tapioca flour

Directions
1. Roughly chop vegetables and potatoes and press garlic. Halve the sugar snap peas.
2. Put the carrots, sweet potatoes and onions in the slow cooker.
3. Mix tapioca flour with curry powder, cumin, chili powder, salt and cinnamon and sprinkle this mixture on the vegetables.
4. Pour the vegetable broth over it.
5. Cover the lid and simmer for 6 hours on a low setting.
6. Stir in the tomatoes and sugar snap peas for the last hour.

Nutrition: 397 Calories 9.35g Protein 6.07g Fat

Fried Cauliflower Rice

Preparation Time: 51 minutes
Cooking Time: 16 minutes
Servings: 2

Ingredients
- 1-piece Cauliflower
- 2 tablespoon Coconut oil
- 1-piece Red onion
- 4 Garlic cloves
- ¼ cup Vegetable broth
- 1.5 cm fresh ginger
- 1 tsp. Chili flakes
- ½ pc. Carrot
- ½ pc. Red bell pepper
- ½ pc. Lemon juice
- 2 tbsp. Pumpkin seeds
- 2 tbsp. fresh coriander

Directions
1. Cut the cauliflower into small rice grains in a food processor.
2. Finely chop the onion, garlic and ginger, cut the carrot into thin strips, dice the bell pepper and finely chop the herbs.
3. Cook 1 tablespoon of coconut oil in a pan and add half of the onion and garlic to the pan and fry briefly until translucent.
4. Add cauliflower rice and season with salt.
5. Pour in the broth and stir everything until it evaporates and the cauliflower rice is tender.
6. Pull rice out of the pan and set it aside.
7. Melt the rest of the coconut oil in the pan and add the remaining onions, garlic, ginger, carrots and peppers.
8. Cook until the vegetables are tender. Sprinkle with a little salt.
9. Add the cauliflower rice again, heat the whole dish and add the lemon juice.
10. Garnish with pumpkin seeds and coriander before serving.

Nutrition: 230 Calories 5.12g Protein 17.8g Fat

Fried Chicken and Broccolini

Preparation time: 10 minutes
Cooking time: 35 minutes
Servings: 2

Ingredients
- 2 tablespoon Coconut oil
- 400 g (14 oz.) Chicken breast
- 150 g (5 ¼ oz.) Bacon cubes
- 250 g (8 oz.) Broccolini

Directions
1. Cut the chicken into cubes.
2. Pre-heat coconut oil in a pan over medium heat and brown the chicken with the bacon cubes and cook through.
3. Season with chili flakes, salt and pepper.
4. Add broccolini and fry.
5. Stack on a plate and enjoy!

Nutrition: 461 Calories 72g Protein 32g Fat

Turkey with Cauliflower Couscous

Preparation Time: 43 minutes
Cooking Time: 12 minutes
Servings: 2

Ingredients
- 150g cauliflower, roughly chopped
- 1 garlic clove, finely chopped
- 40g red onion, finely chopped
- 1 bird's eye chili, finely chopped
- 1 tsp finely chopped fresh ginger
- 2 tbsp extra virgin olive oil
- 2 tsp ground turmeric
- 30g sun dried tomatoes, finely chopped
- 10g parsley
- 150g turkey steak
- 1 tsp dried sage
- Juice of ½ lemon

- 1 tbsp capers

Directions
1. Disintegrate the cauliflower using a food processor. Blend in 1-2 pulses until the cauliflower has a breadcrumb-like consistency.
2. In a skillet, fry garlic, chili, ginger and red onion in 1 tsp olive oil for 3 minutes. Sprinkle in the turmeric and cauliflower then cook for 2 minutes. Remove from heat and add the tomatoes and roughly half the parsley.
3. Garnish the turkey steak with sage and dress with oil. Over medium heat, fry the turkey steak for 6 minutes. Stir in lemon juice, capers and a dash of water then serve with the couscous.

Nutrition: 462 Calories 16.8g Protein 39.9g Fat

Chicken Thighs with Creamy Tomato Spinach Sauce

Preparation Time: 44 minutes
Cooking Time: 13 minutes
Servings: 2

Ingredients
- One tablespoon olive oil
- 1.5 lb. chicken thighs, boneless skinless
- ½ teaspoon salt
- ¼ teaspoon pepper
- 8 oz. tomato sauce
- Two garlic cloves, minced
- ½ cup overwhelming cream
- 4 oz. new spinach
- Four leaves fresh basil (or utilize ¼ teaspoon dried basil)

Directions
1. In a much skillet heat olive oil on medium warmth. Boneless chicken with salt and pepper. Add top side down to the hot skillet.
2. Cook for 5 minutes on medium heat, until the high side, is pleasantly burned. Flip over to the opposite side and heat for five additional minutes on medium heat.
3. Expel the chicken from the skillet to a plate. Step by step instructions to make creamy tomato basil sauce: To the equivalent, presently void skillet, include tomato sauce, minced garlic, substantial cream. Bring to bubble and mix.
4. Lessen warmth to low stew. Include new spinach and new basil. Mix until spinach withers and diminishes in volume.
5. Taste the sauce and include progressively salt and pepper, if necessary. Include back cooked boneless skinless chicken thighs, increment warmth to medium.

Nutrition: 1061 Calories 66g Protein 77g Fat

Sirt Chili with Meat

Preparation Time: 81 minutes
Cooking Time: 63 minutes
Servings: 4

Ingredients
- 1 red onion, finely cleaved
- 3 garlic cloves, finely cleaved
- 2 Bird's Eye chilies, finely hacked
- 1 tbsp additional virgin olive oil
- 1 tbsp ground cumin
- 1 tbsp ground turmeric
- 400g lean minced hamburger (5 percent fat)
- 150ml red wine
- 1 red pepper, cored, seeds evacuated and cut into reduced down pieces
- 2 x 400g tins cleaved tomatoes
- 1 tbsp tomato purée
- 1 tbsp cocoa powder
- 150g tinned kidney beans
- 300ml hamburger stock
- 5g coriander, cleaved
- 5g parsley, cleaved
- 160g buckwheat

Directions
1. Cook onion, garlic and bean stew in the oil over a medium heat for 3 minutes
2. Include the pounded hamburger and dark colored at high heat. Stir in red wine
3. Incorporate red pepper, tomatoes, tomato purée, cocoa, kidney beans and stock and set aside for 60 minutes.
4. Cook the buckwheat and present with the stew.

Nutrition: 346 Calories 14g Protein 11.4g Fat

Chickpea, Quinoa and Turmeric Curry

Preparation Time: 82 minutes
Cooking Time: 1 hour
Servings: 6

Ingredients

- 500g new potatoes, split
- 3 garlic cloves, squashed
- 3 teaspoons ground turmeric
- 1 teaspoon ground coriander
- 1 teaspoon stew drops or powder
- 1 teaspoon ground ginger
- 400g (14 oz.) container of coconut milk
- 1 tbsp tomato purée
- 400g (14 oz.) container of slashed tomatoes
- Salt and pepper
- 180g (6 ¼ oz.) quinoa
- 400g (14 oz.) container of chickpeas, depleted and flushed
- 150g (6 oz.) spinach

Directions

1. Spot the potatoes in a dish of cold water and bring to the boil, at that point let them cook for around 25 minutes
2. Spot the potatoes in an enormous skillet and include the garlic, turmeric, coriander, bean stew, ginger, tomatoes, coconut milk, and tomato purée
3. Boil, season well, stir in quinoa with a cup of simply boil water (300ml - 10 fl. oz.).
4. Diminish the heat to a stew, place the top on and permit to cook. Throughout the following 30 minutes, blending at regular intervals or so to ensure nothing adheres to the base.
5. Halfway through cooking, include the chickpeas. When there are only 5 minutes left, include the spinach and mix it in until it withers. Once the quinoa has cooked and is cushioned, not crunchy, it's prepared.
6. On the off chance that you like a touch of heat, add a cut red bean stew to the cooking curry simultaneously as different flavors.

Nutrition: 609 Calories 23g Protein 22.2g Fat

Chargrilled Beef with a Red Wine

Preparation Time: 18 minutes
Cooking Time: 37 minutes
Servings: 2

Ingredients

- 100 grams potatoes (peeled and cut into 2cm dice)
- 1 tbsp extra virgin olive oil
- 5g parsley, finely chopped
- 50g red onion, sliced into rings
- 50g Kale, sliced
- 1 garlic clove, finely chopped
- 120-150g sirloin steak
- 40ml red wine
- 150ml beef stock
- 1 tsp tomato purée
- 1 tsp corn flour, mix with 1 tbsp water

Directions

1. Heat your oven to (430°F).
2. Situate potatoes in a saucepan with boiling water.
3. Bring back to the boil now cook for 4–5 minutes.
4. Drain.
5. Now place in a roasting tin with 1 teaspoon of the oil. Roast it in the hot oven for about 35 to 45 mins.
6. Turn the potatoes every 10 minutes.
7. When it is cooked, remove from the oven. Then sprinkle with the chopped parsley and mix well.
8. Fry the onion in 1 teaspoon oil and heat for 5 minutes. Fry till they get soft and nicely caramelized. Keep warm. Now steam the Kale for 2–3 minutes then drain.
9. Fry the garlic gently oil (1/2 tablespoon oil). Fry for one minute. It should get soft, but it should not be colored. Add the Kale and fry for 2 minutes more, until it gets tender. Keep warm.
10. Heat a frying pan over high heat. Heat until smoking.
11. Coat the meat in ½ teaspoon of the oil, fry in the hot pan over a medium to high temperature, i.e. heat according to how you like your meat cooked.

12. If you like to cook the meat on a medium level, it would be better to sear the meat. Now transfer the pan to an oven set at 220°C/gas 7(430°F). Finish the cooking that way for a specific time.
13. Remove the meat from the pan. Set aside to rest. Now add the wine to the hot pan to bring up if any meat residue is left. Bubble to reduce the wine by its half. It becomes syrupy with a thick flavor in this way.
14. Add stock and tomato purée to the steak pan to boil it. Then keep adding the corn flour paste to thicken the sauce, adding it a little at a time.
15. Stir in any of the juices from your steak.
16. Serve it with the roasted potatoes, Kale, onion rings and the red wine sauce.

Nutrition: 240 Calories 14.2g Protein 14.4g Fat

Creamy Beef and Shells

Preparation Time: 8 minutes
Cooking Time: 32 minutes
Servings: 3

Ingredients:
- 8 ounces medium pasta shells
- One tablespoon olive oil
- 1-pound ground meat
- One little sweet onion (diced)
- Five cloves garlic (minced)
- One teaspoon Italian flavoring
- One teaspoon dried parsley
- 1/2 teaspoon dried oregano
- Two tablespoons generally useful flour
- 1 cup meat stock
- 1 (15oz can) marinara sauce
- 3/4 cup overwhelming cream
- 1/4 cup sharp cream
- Legitimate salt and crisply ground dark pepper (to taste)
- 1/2 cups cheddar (newly ground)

Directions:
1. Cook pasta as per bundle directions in an enormous pot of bubbling salted water and channel well. W olive oil in a large skillet over medium-high warmth. Include ground meat and cook for 4 minutes.
2. With a same skillet, stir diced onion, and cook for 2minutes. Include garlic, and cook until fragrant, around one moment.
3. Speed in flour until delicately caramelized, for around one moment. Step by step rush in hamburger stock and mix. Incorporate marinara sauce, Italian flavoring, dried parsley, oregano, and paprika.
4. Heat to the boiling point, diminish warmth and stew, mixing once in a while until decreased and somewhat thickened around 6-8 minutes. Mix in cooked pasta, include back meat.
5. Mix in overwhelming cream until warmed through, about 1-2 minutes. Taste and change for salt and pepper. Mix in sour cream. Mix in cheddar until liquefied, about 1-2 minutes. Serve promptly, embellish with parsley whenever wanted.

Nutrition: 624 Calories 63g Fat 40g Protein

Rowdy Enchiladas

Preparation Time: 9 minutes
Cooking Time: 29 minutes
Servings: 3

Ingredients
- Two large chicken breasts (about 400g)
- 2 red peppers, thinly chopped
- 1 tablespoon olive oil
- 3/4 tsp mild chili powder
- 10g fresh coriander, roughly sliced
- For the sauce
- 1 tablespoon olive oil
- 1/2 onion, finely chopped
- 2 tsp cloves, crushed
- 500g tomato passata
- 1 tablespoon chipotle chili paste
- 400g tin black beans drained and rinsed
- 1/2 lime, juiced

Directions:
1. Preheats the oven to gas 5, 190°c, buff 170°c. Set the chicken at a 20 x 30cm skillet with all the peppers olive oil, chili powder, cumin, and paprika. Mix to coat, then cover with foil. Roast for 25-30 mins. Take out the chicken from the dish and then shred with two forks. Reserve in a bowl.

2. Meanwhile, make the sauce. Heat the oil in a saucepan on a low heat and cook the garlic and onion for 10 mins.
3. Stir from the passata and chipotle chili glue; increase heat to moderate, simmer for 10 mins. Bring the beans and carrot juice season.
4. Mix one-third of this sauce plus half of the mozzarella to the cultured broccoli and chicken.
5. To gather, spoon 4 tablespoons of this sauce in exactly the exact baking dish before. Spoon a bit of the chicken mixture down the middle of each tortilla, roll up and then put from the dish.
6. Repeat with the tortillas and filling, then placing them alongside in order that they do not shatter. Scatter together with all the coriander to function.

Nutrition: 674 Calories 57g Fat 37g Protein

Braised Pork Belly and Avocado Skewers

Preparation Time: 12 minutes
Cooking Time: 27 minutes
Servings: 3
Ingredients:
- 1 1/2 pounds pork belly
- One tablespoon samba
- 6 cups of water
- Two tablespoons sugar
- Two tablespoons whole-grain mustard
- 1/2 tablespoon salt
- One teaspoon cayenne
- Three tablespoons sherry vinegar
- Two avocados, cubed
- Eight skewers

Directions:
1. Preheat oven to 300°F. Place samba, water, sugar, mustard, salt, cayenne and sherry vinegar in a small saucepan, heat just until sugar and salt dissolve. Place pork in a baking dish and cover with braising liquid.
2. Cover dish with plastic wrap, followed by aluminum foil. Braise in the oven and cook for approximately 3 1/2 hours, or until tender. Remove pork belly and let cool. While the pork belly is cooling, drain liquid and place in a small saucepot.
3. Reduce until consistency has developed, then remove from heat. Once the abdomen is cold, slice into one 1/2-inch cube. Skewer one piece of pork and one piece of avocado on a skewer. Grill while basting with the sauce and serve.

Nutrition: 599 Calories 54g Fat 32g Protein

Chicken Ayam

Preparation Time: 14 minutes
Cooking Time: 34 minutes
Servings: 3
Ingredients:
- One sliced red chili
- One teaspoon of ginger
- One small red onion, sliced
- One teaspoon turmeric
- One teaspoon galangal
- Four cloves of garlic
- One pinch black pepper
- Three tips muscovado sugar
- Three tsp. shrimp paste
- 1/3 cup coconut milk

Directions:
1. Season the chicken legs. Put on low heat on the grill for about 10 min on one side. Bring all the ingredients together as finely as possible using a mortar and pestle or a blender.
2. Fry in some peanut oil. Put some paste on the chicken. Cook the other side for about 5 min. Add some glue to the chicken.
3. Move to the hotter side of the grill, flip, baste and cook for three additional minutes on both sides. Grill the cake on both sides.

Nutrition: 557 Calories 39g Fat 28g Protein

Sri Lankan-Style Sweet Potato Curry

Preparation Time: 17 minutes
Cooking Time: 39 minutes
Servings: 3
Ingredients
- 1/2 onion, roughly sliced
- 3 garlic cloves, roughly sliced
- 25g sliced ginger, chopped and peeled
- 15g fresh coriander stalks and leaves split leaves sliced

- Two 1/2 tablespoon moderate tikka curry powder
- 60g package cashew nuts
- 1 tablespoon olive oil
- 500g Red Mere farms sweet potatoes, peeled and cut into 3cm balls
- 400ml tin isle sun coconut-milk
- 1/2 vegetable stock block, as much as 300ml
- 200g grower's harvest long-grain rice
- 300g frozen green beans
- 150g Red Mere farms lettuce
- 1 sun trail farms lemon, 1/2 juiced, 1/2 cut into wedges to function

Directions:
1. Set the onion, ginger, garlic, coriander stalks, tikka powder along with half of the cashew nuts in a food processor. Insert 2 tablespoons water and blitz into a chunky paste.
2. In a large skillet, warm the oil over moderate heat. Insert the paste and cook, stirring for 5 mins. Place in the sweet potatoes, stir, then pour into the coconut milk and stock.
3. Bring to the simmer and boil for 25-35 mins before the sweet potatoes are tender.
4. Meanwhile, cook the rice, following packet directions. Toast the rest of the cashews in a dry skillet.
5. Stir the beans into the curry and then simmer for two minutes. Insert the lettuce in handfuls, allowing each to simmer before adding the following; simmer for 1 minute. Drizzle lemon juice and the majority of the coriander leaves.
6. Sprinkle on the remaining coriander and cashews. Serve with the rice and lemon wedges.

Nutrition: 571 Calories 52g Fat 37g Protein

Chicken Liver Along with Tomato Ragu

Preparation Time: 11 minutes
Cooking Time: 27 minutes
Servings: 3

Ingredients
- 2 tablespoon olive oil
- 1 onion, finely chopped
- 2 carrots, scrubbed and simmer
- 4 garlic cloves, finely chopped
- 1/4 x 30g pack fresh ginger, stalks finely chopped, leaves ripped
- 380g package chicken livers, finely chopped,
- 400g tin grower's harvest chopped berries
- 1 chicken stock cube, created around 300ml
- 1/2 tsp caster sugar
- 300g penne
- 1/4 sun trail farms lemon, juiced

Direction:
1. Cook 1 tablespoon oil in a skillet, over a low-medium heating system. Fry the onion and carrots to 10 minutes, stirring periodically. Stir in the ginger and garlic cloves and cook 2 minutes more. Transfer into a bowl set aside.
2. Turn the pan into high heat and then add the oil. Add the chicken livers and simmer for 5 mins until browned. Pour the onion mix to the pan and then stir in the tomatoes, sugar, and stock. Season well, boil, then simmer for 20 mins. Meanwhile, cook pasta to package guidelines.
3. Taste the ragu and put in a second pinch of sugar or more seasoning, if needed. Put in a squeeze of lemon juice to taste and stir in two of the shredded basil leaves. Divide the pasta between four bowls, then spoon across the ragu and top with the rest of the basil.

Nutrition: 497 Calories 39g Fat 21g Protein

Minted Lamb with A Couscous Salad

Preparation Time: 16 minutes
Cooking Time: 32 minutes
Servings: 3

Ingredients
- 75g couscous
- 1/2 chicken stock block, composed to 125ml
- 30g pack refreshing flat-leaf parsley, sliced
- 3 mint sprigs, leaves picked and sliced
- 1 tablespoon olive oil
- 200g pack suspended BBQ minted lamb leg beans, defrosted

- 200g lettuce berries, sliced
- 1/4 tsp, sliced
- 1 spring onion, sliced
- Pinch of ground cumin
- 1/2 lemon, zested and juiced
- 50g reduced-fat salad cheese

Directions:
1. Situate couscous into a heatproof bowl and then pour on the inventory. Cover and set aside for 10 mins, then mash with fork and stir in the herbs.
2. Brush little oil within the lamb steaks and season. Cook to package guidelines, then slit.
3. Blend tomatoes, cucumber and spring onion into the couscous with the oil, the cumin, and lemon juice and zest. Crumble on the salad and serve with the bunny.

Nutrition: 607 Calories 57g Fat 34g Protein

Garbanzo Kale Curry

Preparation Time: 18 minutes
Cooking Time: 41 minutes
Servings 8

Ingredients
- 4 cups dry garbanzo beans
- Curry Paste, but go low on the heat
- 1 cup sliced tomato
- 2 cups kale leaves
- 1/2 cup coconut milk

Directions
1. Put ingredients in the slow cooker. Close & cook on low for 8 hours.

Nutrition: 471 Calories 34g Fat 24g Protein

Buckwheat Kasha with Mushrooms and Onions

Preparation Time: 17 minutes
Cooking Time: 28 minutes
Servings: 3

Ingredients:
- Buckwheat, uncooked – 1 cup
- Olive oil, extra virgin – 3 tablespoons
- Vegetable broth – 2 cups
- Red onion, thinly sliced – 1
- Black ground pepper – .5 teaspoon
- Parsley, chopped – 3 tablespoons
- Walnuts, chopped – 3 tablespoons
- Peas, frozen – 1 cup
- Button mushrooms, sliced – 10 ounces
- Sea salt – 1.5 teaspoons

Directions:
1. On your stove set a medium-sized saucepan and pour the buckwheat and vegetable broth into it, stirring them together. Add in approximately half of the sea salt and black pepper.
2. Allow the broth to come to a boil over medium-high heat before reducing the heat to medium-low and covering the pot with a lid. Continue to cook until the buckwheat is tender. It should cook for an estimated ten minutes more.
3. Meanwhile, while the buckwheat cooks prepare the vegetables. Add the extra virgin olive oil into a favorite large skillet and sauté the onions until tender and slightly golden, about five minutes over medium heat.
4. Put the mushrooms into the hot skillet and continue to heat until the mushrooms are tender and begin to release their juices, about seven minutes. Stir in the peas and remaining seasoning, cooking until the peas are heated through, about three minutes.
5. Add the cooked buckwheat, parsley, and walnuts to the skillet, tossing it all together. Continue to cook the dish together until the flavors meld, about three additional minutes. Serve while warm.

Nutrition: 611 Calories 58g Fat 37g Protein

Sirtfood Cauliflower Couscous & Turkey Steak

Preparation Time: 14 minutes
Cooking Time: 52 minutes
Servings: 4

Ingredients
- 150g cauliflower, roughly chopped
- 1 garlic clove, finely chopped
- 40g red onion, finely chopped
- 1 bird's eye chili, finely chopped
- 1 tsp finely chopped fresh ginger
- 2 tbsp extra virgin olive oil
- 2 tsp ground turmeric
- 30g sun dried tomatoes, finely chopped
- 10g parsley
- 150g turkey steak

- 1 tsp dried sage
- Juice of ½ lemon
- 1 tbsp capers

Directions
1. Disintegrate the cauliflower using a food processor. Blend in 1-2 pulses
2. In a skillet, fry garlic, chili, ginger and red onion in olive oil for 2 minutes. Toss in the turmeric and cauliflower then cook for 1 minute. Remove from heat and add the tomatoes and roughly half the parsley.
3. Garnish the turkey steak with sage and dress with oil. With a skillet, over medium heat, cook turkey steak for 5 minutes. Drizzle lemon juice, capers and a dash of water. Side with the couscous.

Nutrition: 577 Calories 50g Fat 34g Protein

Turkey Escalope with Cauliflower Couscous

Preparation Time: 7 minutes
Cooking Time: 48 minutes
Servings 2

Ingredients
- 150g cauliflower, roughly chopped
- 1 clove of garlic, finely chopped
- 40g red onions, finely chopped
- 1 Thai chili, finely chopped
- 1 teaspoon chopped fresh ginger
- 2 tablespoons of extra virgin olive oil
- 2 teaspoons turmeric
- 30g dried tomatoes, finely chopped
- 10g parsley leaves
- 150g turkey escalope
- 1 teaspoon dried sage
- Juice of a 1/4 lemon
- 1 tablespoon capers

Directions
1. Mix the cauliflower in a food processor until the individual pieces are slightly smaller than a grain of rice.
2. Heat the garlic, onions, chili and ginger in a frying pan with a tablespoon of olive oil until they are slightly glazed. Add turmeric and cauliflower, mix well and heat for about 1 minute. Then remove from heat and add half of the parsley and all the tomatoes and mix well.
3. Mix the turkey escalope with the oil and sage. Put the rest of the oil in a pan and fry the scallops on both sides until they are ready. Then add the lemon juice, capers, remaining parsley and a tablespoon of water and warm it up again briefly. Serve with the cauliflower couscous.

Nutrition: 574 Calories 48g Fat 29g Protein

Tomato & Goat's Cheese Pizza

Preparation Time: 8 minutes
Cooking Time: 51 minutes
Servings 2

Ingredients
- 225g 8oz buckwheat flour
- 2 teaspoons dried yeast
- Pinch of salt
- 150mls 5fl oz slightly water
- 1 teaspoon olive oil

For Topping:
- 75g 3oz feta cheese, crumbled
- 75g 3oz passata or tomato paste
- 1 tomato, sliced
- 1 red onion, finely chopped
- 25g 1oz rocket arugula leaves, chopped
- 562 calories per serving

Directions
1. Incorporate all the ingredients for the pizza dough then allow it to stand for 60 minutes
2. Roll the dough out to a size to suit you. Spoon the passata onto the base and add the rest of the toppings.
3. Bake at 400F for 18 minutes and serve.

Nutrition: 604 Calories 59g Fat 33g Protein

Roast Duck Legs with Red Wine Sauce

Preparation Time: 12 minutes
Cooking Time: 64 minutes
Servings: 3

Ingredients
- 1 bunch fresh rosemary, chopped
- 4 large garlic cloves
- 4 duck legs
- Salt to taste
- 1 teaspoon Chinese five-spice powder
- 1 ½ cups red wine
- 1 ½ tablespoons red currant jelly

Directions
1. Preheat an oven to 375 degrees.
2. Spread the rosemary sprigs and whole garlic cloves in a 9x13-inch baking dish.
3. Situate duck legs on top of the rosemary, and season with salt and five-spice powder. Bake for 1 hour.
4. Boil wine over medium-high heat. Once cooked, pour off and discard the fat. Drizzle the wine sauce over the duck legs and bake 17 minutes.

Nutrition: 607 Calories 54g Fat 31g Protein

Arugula-Stuffed Steak

Preparation Time: 13 minutes
Cooking Time: 72 minutes
Servings: 3

Ingredients
- 1 cup baby arugula
- 1 jar roasted red peppers
- 1 egg white
- ½ cup seasoned breadcrumbs
- ¼ cup Parmesan, grated
- ¼ cup sunflower seeds, toasted
- 1 garlic clove, minced
- Salt and pepper to taste
- 1 ½ -pound flank steak

Directions
1. Preheat oven to 350 degrees F.
2. Mix arugula with the roasted red peppers, egg white, breadcrumbs, Parmesan, sunflower seeds, minced garlic and salt and pepper to taste.
3. Cut the flank steak horizontally along the long edge to within ½" of the opposite edge.
4. Open your steak and use a meat mallet to flatten to ½" thickness.
5. Spread arugula mixture over the steak to within 1" of the edges.
6. Roll like a jelly roll, starting with a long side. Tie with some kitchen string and place in a greased 13-in. x 9-in. x 2-in. baking dish.
7. Cover and bake for 60 minutes
8. Uncover and bake for 42 minutes
9. Let stand for 13 minutes and cut into ½" slices to serve.

Nutrition: 551 Calories 53g Fat 30g Protein

Beef Stroganoff French Bread Toast

Preparation Time: 9 minutes
Cooking Time: 52 minutes
Servings: 3

Ingredient:
- Four tablespoons olive oil
- 1/2 cups mushrooms
- Two teaspoons salt, separated
- 1/2 teaspoon dark pepper
- Two tablespoons thyme
- Two tablespoons spread
- 1/2 cup onions, diced
- Two cloves garlic, minced
- 1-pound ground meat
- Three tablespoons generally useful flour
- Two teaspoons paprika
- 1/2 cups meat juices
- 1/2 cup sharp cream
- One teaspoon Dijon mustard

For the toasts:
- One portion French bread, inner parts dugout
- 2 cups mozzarella
- Three tablespoons cleaved Italian parsley

Directions:
1. Preheat stove to 350 degrees, and line a sheet container with material paper. Make the stroganoff: In a large Dutch grill or skillet, heat olive oil over medium warmth. Sauté mushrooms with one teaspoon salt and dark pepper. Include thyme.
2. Cook mushrooms until brilliant, roughly 4 minutes. Expel from a dish and put in a safe spot. Include margarine, onions and garlic to the container and sauté 2 minutes. Cook ground hamburger over medium warmth until dark-colored, roughly 4 minutes.
3. Add flour and paprika to cover uniformly. Include meat soup, sour cream and mustard. Blend entirely and include mushrooms back in. Round the emptied portion with stroganoff and top with mozzarella cheddar.
4. Spot on the readied heating sheet and prepare for 5 to 10 minutes until cheddar is

brilliant and softened. Head with parsley, cut and serve right away.

Nutrition: 615 Calories 61g Fat 37g Protein

Beef Burritos

Preparation Time: 12 minutes
Cooking Time: 23 minutes
Servings: 6

Ingredients:

- ¼ cup white onion, chopped
- ¼ cup green bell pepper, chopped
- 1-pound ground beef
- ¼ cup tomato puree, low-sodium
- ¼ teaspoon ground black pepper
- ¼ teaspoon ground cumin
- 6 flour tortillas, burrito size

Directions:

1. Take a skillet pan, place it over medium heat and when hot, add beef and cook for 5 to 8 minutes until browned.
2. Drain the excess fat, then transfer beef to a plate lined with paper towels and serve.
3. Return pan over medium heat, grease it with oil and when hot, add pepper and onion and cook for 4 minutes.
4. Switch to low heat, return beef to the pan, season with black pepper and cumin, pour in tomato puree, stir until mixed and cook for 5 minutes until done.
5. Lay beef mixture evenly on top of the tortilla, roll them in burrito style by folding both ends and then serve.

Nutrition: 265 Calories 9g Fat 15g Protein

Meatballs with Eggplant

Preparation Time: 17 minutes
Cooking Time: 63 minutes
Servings: 6

Ingredients:

- 1-pound ground beef
- ½ cup green bell pepper, chopped
- 2 medium eggplants, peeled and diced
- ½ teaspoon minced garlic
- 1 cup stewed tomatoes
- ½ cup white onion, diced
- 1/3 cup canola oil
- 1 teaspoon lemon and pepper seasoning, salt-free
- 1 teaspoon turmeric
- 1 teaspoon Mrs. Dash seasoning blend
- 2 cups of water

Directions:

1. Take a large skillet pan, place it over medium heat, add oil in it and when hot, add garlic and green bell pepper and cook for 4 minutes until sauté.
2. Transfer green pepper mixture to a plate, set aside until needed then eggplant pieces into the pan and cook for 8 minutes on both sides and set aside until needed.
3. Take a medium bowl, place beef in it, add onion, season with all the spices, stir then shape the mix into 30 small meatballs.
4. Place meatballs into the pan in a single layer and cook for 3 minutes, or until browned.
5. When done, place all the meatballs in the pan, add cooked bell pepper mixture in it along with eggplant, stir in water and tomatoes and simmer for 30 minutes at low heat setting until thoroughly cooked.
6. Serve straight away.

Nutrition: 265 Calories 18g Fat 17g Protein

Slow-Cooked Lemon Chicken

Preparation Time: 24 minutes
Cooking Time: 7 hours
Servings: 4

Ingredients:

- 1 teaspoon dried oregano
- ¼ teaspoon ground black pepper
- 2 tablespoons butter, unsalted
- 1-pound chicken breast, boneless, skinless
- ¼ cup chicken broth, low sodium
- ¼ cup water
- 1 tablespoon lemon juice
- 2 cloves garlic, minced
- 1 teaspoon fresh basil, chopped

Direction:

1. Blend oregano and ground black pepper. Brush mix over the chicken.
2. Cook butter in a medium-sized skillet at medium heat. Stir in chicken then transfer to the slow cooker.
3. Boil chicken broth, water, lemon juice and garlic in the skillet. Pour over the chicken.

4. Cover, adjust slow cooker at low for 5 hours.
5. Mix basil and baste chicken. Cover, cook at high for an additional 15–30 minutes

Nutrition: 197 Calories 9g Fat 26g Protein

Smothered Pork Chops and Sautéed Greens

Preparation Time: 23 minutes
Cooking Time: 61 minutes
Servings: 6

Ingredients:
Smothered Pork Chops:
- 6 pork loin chops
- 1 tbsp. black pepper
- 2 tsp. Paprika
- 2 tsp. granulated onion powder
- 2 tsp. granulated garlic powder
- 1 cup and 2 tbsp. flour
- ½ cup canola oil
- 2 cups low-sodium beef stock
- 1 ½ cups fresh onions, sliced
- ½ cup fresh scallions, sliced on the bias

Sautéed Greens:
- 8 cups fresh collard greens, chopped and blanched
- 2 tablespoons olive oil
- 1 tablespoon unsalted butter
- ¼ cup onions, finely diced
- 1 tablespoon fresh garlic, chopped
- 1 teaspoon crushed red pepper flakes
- 1 teaspoon black pepper
- 1 teaspoon vinegar (optional)

Direction:
1. Set oven to 350° F.

Pork Chops:
2. Incorporate black pepper, paprika, onion powder and garlic powder. With a half of mixture, rub with both sides of the pork chops then use the other half with 1 cup flour.
3. Set aside 2 tablespoons of flour mix.
4. Slightly coat pork chops with seasoned flour.
5. Cook oil in oven-ready sauté pan over medium-high.
6. Cook pork chops for 6 minutes on both sides. Take out from pan
7. Cook onions for 5 minutes. Mix 2 tablespoons of reserved flour with onions for about 1 minute.
8. Gradually, add beef stock and stir until thickened.
9. Place pork chops to pan and coat with sauce. Seal with foil and cook for 45 minutes at 350° F.
10. Take out from oven and cool for 8 minutes before serving.

Sautéed Greens:
11. To blanch greens, place greens to a boiling water for 30 seconds.
12. Drain boiling water off and quickly transfer in a bowl of ice and water.
13. Cool then drain and set aside.
14. In large sauté pan on medium-high heat, cook butter and oil together. Sauté onions and garlic for 6 minutes.
15. Cook collard greens and black and red pepper for 7 minutes on high heat.
16. Pull out from heat; stir in vinegar if desired.

Nutrition: 464 Calories 28g Fat 27g Protein

Pasta with Cheesy Meat Sauce

Preparation Time: 17 minutes
Cooking Time: 26 minutes
Servings: 6

Ingredients:
- ½ box large-shaped pasta
- 1-pound ground beef
- ½ cup onions
- 1 tbsp. onion flakes
- 1½ cups beef stock
- 1 tbsp. Better Than Bouillon® beef
- 1 tablespoon tomato sauce, no salt added
- ¾ cup Monterey or pepper jack cheese, shredded
- 8 ounces cream cheese, softened
- ½ teaspoon Italian seasoning
- ½ teaspoon ground black pepper
- 2 tablespoons French's® Worcestershire sauce, reduced sodium

Direction
1. Cook pasta noodles following the directions on the box.

2. In a sauté pan, fry ground beef, onions and onion flakes until the meat is browned.
3. Strain and add stock, bouillon and tomato sauce.
4. Simmer, stirring occasionally. Put in cooked pasta, turn off heat, and mix softened cream cheese, shredded cheese and seasonings. Stir pasta mixture.

Nutrition: 502 Calories 30g Fat 23g Protein

Aromatic Herbed Rice

Preparation Time: 14 minutes
Cooking Time: 18 minutes
Servings: 6

Ingredients:
- 2 tablespoons olive oil
- 3 cups cooked rice (don't overcook)
- 4–5 cloves fresh garlic, sliced thin
- 2 tablespoons fresh cilantro, chopped
- 2 tablespoons fresh oregano, chopped
- 2 tablespoons fresh chives, chopped
- ½ teaspoon red pepper flakes
- 1 teaspoon red wine vinegar

Directions:
1. In a large sauté pan, heat olive oil on medium-high heat and lightly sauté garlic. Add rice, herbs and red pepper flakes and continue to cook for 2–4 minutes or until well-mixed.
2. Turn off heat, add vinegar, mix well and serve.

Nutrition: 134 Calories 5g Fat 2g Protein

Herb-Crusted Roast Leg of Lamb

Preparation Time: 17 minutes
Cooking Time: 38 minutes
Servings: 12

Ingredients:
- 1 4-pound leg of lamb
- 3 tablespoons lemon juice
- 1 tablespoon curry powder
- 2 cloves garlic, minced
- ½ teaspoon ground black pepper
- 1 cup onions, sliced
- ½ cup dry vermouth

Direction:
1. Prep oven to 400° F.
2. Situate leg of lamb on a roasting pan. Drizzle 1 tsp. of lemon juice.
3. Blend 2 teaspoons of lemon juice and the rest of the spices. Brush paste onto the lamb.
4. Roast lamb at 400° F for 30 minutes.
5. Strain off fat and stir vermouth and onions.
6. Set heat to 325° F and cook for 2 hours. Baste leg of lamb frequently. Pull out from oven and rest 3 minutes before serving.

Nutrition: 292 Calories 20g Fat 24g Protein

Baked Potatoes with Spicy Chickpea

Preparation Time: 18 minutes
Cooking Time: 9 minutes
Servings: 5

Ingredients:
- 4-6 baking potatoes, pricked all over
- Two tablespoons olive oil
- Two red onions, finely chopped
- Four cloves garlic, grated or crushed
- 2cm ginger, grated
- Two tablespoons turmeric
- ½ -2 teaspoons of chili flakes (depending on how hot you like things)
- Two tablespoons cumin seeds
- Splash of water
- Two into 400g tins chopped tomatoes
- Two tablespoons unsweetened cocoa powder (or cacao)
- Two into 400g tins chickpeas (or kidney beans if you prefer) including the chickpea water
- Two yellow peppers (or whatever color you prefer!), chopped into bite size pieces
- Salt and pepper to taste (optional)
- Side salad (optional)

Directions:
1. Preheat the oven to 200C so you can make all the ingredients you need.
2. Put your baking potatoes in the oven when the oven is hot enough, and cook them for an hour or till they are cooked as you want them.
3. Put the olive oil and chopped red onion in a big broad saucepan once the potatoes are in the oven and cook gently with the lid

until the onions are soft but not brown for 5 minutes.
4. Remove the lid and add the garlic, cumin, ginger and chili. Cook on low heat for another minute, and then you add the turmeric and a tiny drizzle of water and cook for 3 minutes, keeping in minute not to let the saucepan get too dry.
5. Add cocoa (or cacao) powder, chickpeas (including chickpea water) and yellow pepper in the tomatoes. Boil it and simmer for 45 minutes at low heat until the sauce is thick and greasy (but don't let it burn!). Stew will be handled roughly at the same time as the potatoes.
6. At last, mix in the two tablespoons of parsley and some salt and pepper, if desired, and serve the stew over the baked potatoes, maybe with a small side salad.

Nutrition: 243 Calories 24g Fat 16g Protein

Buckwheat with Red Onion Dal

Preparation Time: 8 minutes
Cooking Time: 0 minutes
Servings: 4

Ingredients:
- One tablespoon olive oil
- One small red onion, sliced
- Three garlic cloves, grated or crushed
- One bird eye chili deseeded and finely chopped (more if you like things hot!)
- 2 cm ginger, grated
- Two teaspoons turmeric
- Two teaspoons graham masala
- 160g red lentils
- 200ml water
- 400ml coconut milk
- 160g buckwheat (or brown rice)
- 100g kale

Directions:
1. In a big, deep saucepan, put the olive oil and add the sliced onion. Cook at low pressure, with the lid on until softened for 5 minutes.
2. Add the garlic, chili and ginger and cook for 1 minute.
3. Add the turmeric, graham masala, sprinkle with water and cook for 1 minute.
4. Add the red lentils, coconut milk and 200 ml of water (fill the coconut milk with water and drop it into the casserole).
5. Thoroughly mix everything and cook over a gentle heat for 20 minutes with the lid on. If the dhal starts sticking, stir periodically and add a little more water.
6. After 20 minutes, add the Kale, whisk thoroughly and remove the lid and cook for another 5 minutes (1-2 minutes if spinach is used instead!)
7. Place the buckwheat in a medium saucepan about 15 minutes before the curry is ready, and put plenty of boiling water. Bring the water again to the boil and cook for 10 minutes

Nutrition: 234 Calories 19g fat 9g protein

Aromatic Chicken

Preparation Time: 19 minutes
Cooking Time: 13 minutes
Servings: 1

Ingredients:
For the salsa
- One large tomato
- One bird's eye chili, finely chopped
- 1tbsp capers, finely chopped
- 5g parsley, finely chopped
- Juice 1/2 lemon

For the chicken
- 120g skinless, boneless chicken breast
- 2tsp ground turmeric
- Juice 1/2 lemon
- 1tbsp extra virgin olive oil
- 50g kale, chopped
- 20g red onion, sliced
- 1tsp fresh ginger, finely chopped
- 50g buckwheat

Directions:
1. Heat the oven at 220oC/200oC fan/gas level 7
2. Cut the tomato thinly to make the salsa and make sure you hold as much of the liquid as possible. Mix with the chili, capers, lemon juice and parsley.
3. Marinate the chicken breast for 5-10 minutes with 1tsp of turmeric, lemon juice and half of the butter.

4. Heat the frying pan ovenproof; add the marinated chicken and cook each side for a minute until golden, then move to the oven for 8-10 minutes or until cooked through. Remove and cover with tape, then leave for 5 minutes to rest.
5. Then you cook the Kale in a 5-minutesute steamer. In the remaining oil, fry the onion and ginger until soft but not white, then put the cooked Kale and fry for one more minute.
6. Cook the buckwheat with the remaining turmeric as directed, and then serve.

Nutrition: 213 Calories 28g Fat 16g Protein

Fragrant Asian hotpot-Sirtfood

Preparation Time: 13 minutes
Cooking Time: 17 minutes
Servings: 2
Ingredients:
- 1 tsp tomato purée,
- 1-star anise, crushed (or 1/4 tsp ground anise),
- Small handful (10g) parsley, stalks finely chopped,
- Small handful (10g) coriander, stalks finely chopped,
- Juice of 1/2 lime,
- 500ml chicken stock, fresh or made with one cube
- 50 g broccoli, cut into small florets,
- 50 g beans sprout,
- 100g raw tiger prawns,
- 100g firm tofu, chopped,
- 50 g rice noodles, cooked according to packet directions,
- 50 g cooked water chestnuts, drained,
- 20 g sushi ginger, cut

Directions:
1. Stir in the cabbage, broccoli, prawns, tofu, noodles and water chestnuts and cook gently until the prawns are finished. Remove from heat and mix in the ginger sushi and the paste miso.
2. Serve sprinkled with the leaves of the parsley and coriander.

Nutrition: 185 calories 27g Fat 13g Protein

Buckwheat Bean Risotto

Preparation Time: 9 minutes
Cooking Time: 12 minutes
Servings: 2
Ingredients:
- 2 tbsp. of olive oil or butter,
- Two cloves of garlic, minced,
- 225g/8 of buckwheat,
- 400ml of hot water or vegetable stock,
- 225g/8 of frozen broad beans,
- 1/2 cup of sun-dried tomatoes in milk,
- Juice of half a lemon,
- 2 tbsp. of basil or coriander, chopped,
- 50g/2 oz. almonds, toasted, salt, and pepper,

Directions:
1. Cook olive oil in a frying pan. Cook the garlic for one minute.
2. Stir buckwheat to the saucepan and mix well to coat in the butter.
3. Add the stock or hot water. Cover for 10 minutes, and then simmer.
4. Stir in the beans. Cook until the beans are moist, for a few minutes.
5. Season well and stir sun-dried tomatoes, lemon juice, fresh herbs, and almonds.

Nutrition: 389 calories 19g Fat6g Protein

Butterbean and Vegetable

Preparation Time: 17 minutes
Cooking Time: 13 minutes
Servings: 2
Ingredients:
- 3 tbsp. of coconut oil or olive oil,
- One big onion, finely chopped,
- 2 tsp of root ginger, finely chopped,
- One clove of garlic, finely chopped,
- 1-2 tbsp. of curry powder,
- 200g/7 of green beans cut into 2 cm pieces,
- One cauliflower, cut into florets,
- Three sweet potatoes, peeled and chopped into large chunks,
- Two cans of butterbeans (or prepare your using 225g/8 of dried beans),
- 50-100g/2-4 of creamed coconut,
- 1 tbsp. Cook the onions until they are tender.

Directions:
1. Sauté garlic and ginger to the onions.
2. Then throw the green beans, cauliflower, and sweet potatoes into the curry powder and mix well to cover in the spices.
3. Attach the butter beans drained and rinsed, and enough hot water to cover the ingredients. Move some of the liquid from the pan into the bowl and dissolve the coconut cream inside. Remove this to the saucepan and cook for several minutes.
4. Just before serving, sprinkle over the fresh coriander.

Nutrition: 230 calories 31g fat 16g Protein

Lemon Paprika Chicken with Vegetable

Preparation Time: 18 minutes
Cooking Time: 9 minutes
Servings: 2

Ingredients:
- 3 tbsp. of olive oil,
- 2 tbsp. of paprika,
- Two carrots, chopped,
- 1/2 celeriac, peeled and chopped,
- Three turnips, peeled and chopped,
- 300 g of chicken wings,
- 1 pint of hot stock, Sprigs of rosemary and thyme,
- Two bay leaves, salt, and pepper,
- One lemon juice,
- A big bunch of kale, chopped,

Directions:
1. Cook oil in a big pan with a tight lid. Add the paprika, potatoes, celeriac, chicken and turnip wings to the pan and cook for a few minutes.
2. Stir in the pan the stock, spices, salt, pepper, and lemon juice and bring to the boil.
3. Turn the heat down, cover it with a lid, and gently simmer for 40 minutes.
4. Attach the kale and cook until the kale and the chicken are both cooked for a few more minutes.

Nutrition: 321 calories 30g Fat 24g Protein

Spicy Ras-El-Hanout Dressing

Preparation Time: 13 minutes
Cooking Time: 1 minute
Servings: 16

Ingredients:
- 125 ml Olive oil
- 1-piece Lemon (the juice)
- 2 teaspoons Honey
- 1 ½ teaspoons Ras el Hanout
- 1/2 pieces Red pepper

Directions:
1. Remove the seeds from the chili pepper.
2. Chop the chili pepper as finely as possible.
3. Place the pepper in a bowl with lemon juice, honey, and Ras-El-Hanout and whisk with a whisk.
4. Pour olive oil drop by drop while continuing to whisk.

Nutrition: 73 Calories 8g Fats 1g Carbohydrates

Broccoli & Mushroom Chicken

Preparation Time: 13 minutes
Cooking Time: 29 minutes
Servings: 5

Ingredients
- 3 tbsp. olive oil
- 1-pound chicken breast, cubed
- 1 medium onion
- 6 garlic cloves
- 2 cups fresh mushrooms
- 16 oz. broccoli florets
- ¼ cup water

Direction
1. Cook oil in a large wok over medium heat and fry chicken cubes for 4 minutes.
2. Situate chicken cubes onto a plate.
3. In the same wok, sauté onion for 4 minutes.
4. Cook mushrooms for 5 minutes.
5. Mix in the cooked chicken, broccoli, and water, and cook for 9 minutes, stirring occasionally.
6. Season well and remove from heat.

Nutrition: 196 Calories 11g Fat 21g Protein

Beef with Kale & Carrot

Preparation Time: 16 minutes
Cooking Time: 11 minutes
Servings: 4

Ingredients
- 2 tablespoons coconut oil

- 4 garlic cloves, minced
- 1-pound beef sirloin steak, cut into bite-sized pieces
- Ground black pepper, to taste
- 1½ cups carrots, peeled and cut into matchsticks
- 1½ cups fresh kale, tough ribs removed and chopped
- 3 tablespoons tamari

Direction
1. Melt the coconut oil in a wok over medium heat and sauté the garlic for about 1 minute.
2. Add the beef and black pepper and stir to combine.
3. Increase the heat to medium-high and cook for about 3–4 minutes or until browned from all sides.
4. Add the carrot, kale, and tamari, and cook for about 4–5 minutes.
5. Remove from the heat and serve hot.

Nutrition: 311 Calories 13.8g Fat 37g Protein

Lamb Chops with Kale

Preparation Time: 14 minutes
Cooking Time: 13 minutes
Servings: 4

Ingredients
- 1 garlic clove, minced
- 1 tablespoon fresh rosemary leaves, minced
- Salt and ground black pepper, to taste
- 4 lamb loin chops
- 4 cups fresh baby kale

Direction
1. Preheat the grill to high heat. Grease the grill grate.
2. In a bowl, add the garlic, rosemary, salt, and black pepper, and mix well.
3. Coat the lamb chops with the herb mixture generously.
4. Place the chops onto the hot side of grill and cook for about 2 minutes per side.
5. Now, move the chops onto the cooler side of the grill and cook for about 6–7 minutes.
6. Divide the kale onto serving plates and top each with 1 chop and serve.

Nutrition: 301 Calories 10g Fat 42g Protein

Chickpea with Swiss Chard

Preparation Time: 17 minutes
Cooking Time: 12 minutes
Servings: 4

Ingredients
- 2 tablespoon olive oil
- 2 garlic cloves, sliced thinly
- 1 large tomato, chopped finely
- 2 bunches fresh Swiss chard, trimmed
- 1 (18-ounce) can chickpeas, drained and rinsed
- Salt and ground black pepper, to taste
- ¼ cup water
- 1 tablespoon fresh lemon juice
- 2 tablespoons fresh parsley, chopped

Direction
1. Heat the oil in a big wok at medium heat and cook the garlic.
2. Add the tomato and cook for about 2–3 minutes, crushing with the back of spoon.
3. Cook remaining ingredients except lemon juice and parsley for 6 minutes.
4. Drizzle with the lemon juice and remove from the heat.
5. Serve hot with the garnishing of parsley.

Nutrition: 217 Calories 8.3g Fat 8.8g Protein

Tofu & Broccoli Curry

Preparation Time: 21 minutes
Cooking Time: 34 minutes
Servings: 5

Ingredients
- 1 (16-ounce) block firm tofu, drained, pressed, and cut into ½-inch cubes
- 2 tablespoons coconut oil
- 1 medium yellow onion, chopped
- 1½ tablespoons fresh ginger, minced
- 2 garlic cloves, minced
- 1 tablespoon curry powder
- Salt and ground black pepper, to taste
- 1 cup fresh mushrooms, sliced
- 1 cup carrots, peeled and sliced
- 1 (14-ounce) can unsweetened low-fat coconut milk
- ½ cup low-sodium vegetable broth
- 2 teaspoons light brown sugar
- 10 ounces broccoli florets
- 1 tablespoon fresh lime juice

- ¼ cup fresh basil leaves, sliced thinly

Direction
1. In a Dutch oven, cook oil over medium heat and sauté the onion, ginger and garlic for about 5 minutes.
2. Stir in the curry powder, salt, and black pepper, and cook for about 2 minutes, stirring occasionally.
3. Cook mushrooms and carrot for 4 minutes.
4. Stir in the coconut milk, broth, and brown sugar, and bring to a boil.
5. Add the tofu and broccoli and simmer for about 12–15 minutes, stirring occasionally.
6. Drizzle lime juice and remove from the heat.
7. Serve hot.

Nutrition: 184 Calories 11g Fat 10.5g Protein

Chicken & Veggies with Buckwheat Noodles

Preparation Time: 24 minutes
Cooking Time: 22 minutes
Servings: 2

Ingredients
- ½ cup broccoli florets
- ½ cup fresh green beans, trimmed and sliced
- 1 cup fresh kale, tough ribs removed and chopped
- 5 ounces buckwheat noodles
- 1 tablespoon coconut oil
- 1 brown onion, chopped finely
- 1 (6-ounce) boneless, skinless chicken breast, cubed
- 2 garlic cloves, chopped finely
- 3 tablespoons low-sodium soy sauce

Direction
1. In a medium pan of the boiling water, add the broccoli and green beans and cook for about 4–5 minutes.
2. Add the kale and cook for about 1–2 minutes.
3. Drain the vegetables and transfer into a large bowl. Set aside.
4. In another pan of the lightly salted boiling water, cook the soba noodles for about 5 minutes.
5. Drain the noodles well and then, rinse under cold running water. Set aside.
6. Meanwhile, in a large wok, melt the coconut oil over medium heat and sauté the onion for about 2–3 minutes.
7. Cook chicken cubes for 6 minutes.
8. Cook garlic, soy sauce and a little splash of water for 3 minutes, stirring frequently.
9. Add the cooked vegetables and noodles and cook for about 1–2 minutes, tossing frequently.
10. Serve hot with the garnishing of sesame seeds.

Nutrition: 463 Calories 11.7g Fat 22.5g Protein

Veggie Burgers

Preparation Time: 23 minutes
Cooking Time: 8 minutes
Servings: 4

Ingredients
- 1 cup water
- 1/3 cup dry couscous
- 1½ cups broccoli florets
- 2 teaspoons olive oil
- ½ cup onion, chopped
- ½ cup scallion, chopped
- 2 teaspoons ground cumin
- ¼ teaspoon ground turmeric
- 1 tablespoon sesame tahini
- 1 (15-ounce) can chickpeas, rinsed and drained
- ½ cup panko breadcrumbs
- 4 cups fresh kale, tough ribs removed and chopped

Direction
1. Preheat your oven to 400°F. Line a baking sheet with foil paper.
2. In a small pan, mix together water and couscous over medium heat and boil.
3. Pull out from heat and keep aside, covered for about 10 minutes
4. Meanwhile, in a pan of boiling water, arrange a steamer basket.
5. Place the broccoli in steamer basket and steam, covered for about 5–7 minutes.
6. Drain the broccoli well.
7. Using a wok, cook oil over medium heat and sauté the onion and scallion for 4 minutes.

8. Stir in the cumin and turmeric and remove from heat.
9. In a food processor, add the couscous, broccoli, onion mixture, tahini, and chickpeas, and pulse until well combined.
10. Transfer the mixture into a bowl.
11. Add the breadcrumbs and stir to combine.
12. Make equal-sized patties from mixture.
13. Arrange the patties onto the prepared baking sheet in a single layer.
14. Bake for about 50 minutes, flipping once halfway through.
15. Divide kale
16. Top with 1 patty and serve.

Nutrition: 321 Calories 7g Fat 12.8g Protein

Kale with Pine Nuts

Preparation Time: 13 minutes
Cooking Time: 14 minutes
Servings: 4

Ingredients

- 1 tablespoon olive oil
- 2 garlic cloves, minced
- 1½ pounds fresh kale, tough ribs removed and chopped
- ¼ cup water
- 3 teaspoons red wine vinegar
- Salt and ground black pepper, to taste
- 2 tablespoons pine nuts

Direction

1. Heat the olive oil in wok in medium heat and sauté the garlic.
2. Add kale and cook for about 3–4 minutes.
3. Add the water, vinegar, salt, and black pepper, and cook for 4–5 minutes.
4. Remove from heat and stir in the pine nuts.
5. Serve immediately.

Nutrition: 146 Calories 6.5g Fat 5.8g Protein

Bok Choy & Mushroom Stir Fry

Preparation Time: 17 minutes
Cooking Time: 9 minutes
Servings: 4

Ingredients

- 1-pound baby bok choy
- 4 teaspoons olive oil
- 1 teaspoon fresh ginger, minced
- 2 garlic cloves, chopped
- 5 ounces fresh mushrooms, sliced
- 2 tablespoons red wine
- 2 tablespoons soy sauce

Direction

1. Trim bases of bok choy and separate outer leaves from stalks, leaving the smallest inner leaves attached.
2. In a large cast-iron wok, heat the oil over medium-high heat and sauté the ginger and garlic for about 1 minute.
3. Cook mushrooms for 4 minutes, stirring frequently.
4. Stir in the bok choy leaves and stalks and cook for about 1 minute, tossing with tongs.
5. Stir in the wine, soy sauce, and black pepper, and cook for about 2–3 minutes, tossing occasionally.
6. Serve hot.

Nutrition: 77 Calories 5g Fat 3.5g Protein

Prawns with Asparagus

Preparation Time: 16 minutes
Cooking Time: 13 minutes
Servings: 4

Ingredients

- 3 tablespoons olive oil
- 1-pound prawns, peeled, and deveined
- 1-pound asparagus, trimmed
- Salt and ground black pepper, to taste
- 1 teaspoon garlic, minced
- 1 teaspoon fresh ginger, minced
- 1 tablespoon low-sodium soy sauce
- 2 tablespoons lemon juice

Direction

1. In a wok, pre-heat2 tablespoons of oil over medium-high heat and cook the prawns with salt and black pepper for about 3–4 minutes.
2. With a slotted spoon, situate prawns into a bowl. Set aside.
3. In the same wok, heat remaining 1 tablespoon of oil over medium-high heat and cook the asparagus, ginger, garlic, salt, and black pepper and sauté for about 6–8 minutes, stirring frequently.
4. Stir in the prawns and soy sauce and cook for about 1 minute.
5. Pour lemon juice and remove from the heat.

6. Serve hot.

Nutrition: 253 Calories 12.7g Fat 28.7g Protein

SIDES RECIPES

Eggplant Dipped Roasted Asparagus

Preparation Time: 14 minutes
Cooking Time: 35 minutes
Servings: 2

Ingredients

- 4 tbsp olive oil
- ½ pounds asparagus spears, trimmed
- Sea salt and black pepper to taste
- ½ tsp sweet paprika

For Eggplant Dip

- ½ pound eggplants
- 2 tsp olive oil
- ½ cup scallions, chopped
- 2 cloves garlic, minced
- 1 tbsp lemon juice
- ½ tsp chili pepper
- Salt and black pepper, to taste
- Fresh parsley, chopped for garnish

Directions

1. Line a parchment paper to a baking sheet. Add asparagus spears to the baking sheet. Toss with oil, sweet paprika, black pepper, and salt. Bake for 9 minutes at 390°F.
2. Add eggplants on a lined cookie sheet. Position under the broiler for about 20 minutes at 425°F; let the eggplants to cool. Peel them and discard the stems. Situate frying pan over medium-high heat and warm olive oil. Add in garlic and onion; sauté until tender.
3. Using a food processor, pulse together black pepper, roasted eggplants, salt, lemon juice, scallion mixture, and chili pepper to mix evenly.
4. Add parsley for garnishing. Serve alongside roasted asparagus spears.

Nutrition: 169 Calories 12g Fat 5g Protein

Steamed Asparagus & Grilled Cauliflower Steaks

Preparation Time: 13 minutes
Cooking Time: 21 minutes
Servings: 4

Ingredients

- 4 tbsp olive oil
- 1 head cauliflower, sliced into 'steaks'
- 1 red onion, sliced
- ¼ cup green chili sauce
- 1 tsp harissa powder
- Salt and black pepper to taste
- 1 lb. asparagus, trimmed
- Juice of 1 lemon
- 1 cup water
- Fresh parsley to garnish

Directions

1. Preheat the grill.
2. Blend olive oil, chili sauce, and harissa. Brush the cauliflower with the mixture. Situate steaks on the grill, and cook for 6 minutes. Flip the cauliflower, grill further for 6 minutes.
3. Boil water over high heat, place the asparagus in a sieve, and set over the steam from the boiling water. Cook for 6 minutes. After, remove to a bowl and toss with lemon juice. Remove the grilled cauliflower to a plate; sprinkle with salt, black pepper, red onion, and parsley. Serve with the steamed asparagus.

Nutrition: 118 Calories 9g Fat 2g Protein

Endive with Cheddar & Walnut Sauce

Preparation Time: 13 minutes
Cooking Time: 17 minutes
Serving: 2

Ingredients

- 1 endive heads, leaves separated
- 2 oz cheddar cheese, crumbled
- 1 cup heavy cream
- ½ tsp nutmeg
- Salt and black pepper to taste
- ½ cup toasted walnuts

Directions

1. Using a saucepan on medium heat, warm up heavy cream. Add in cheddar cheese, nutmeg, salt, and pepper and stir.
2. Remove to a bowl and whisk with a mixer until smooth. Let cool. Arrange the endive leaves on a serving plate.

3. Spoon the cheese mixture into the leaves and top with toasted walnuts to serve.

Nutrition: 360 Calories 23g Fat 12g Protein

Asian-Style Tofu Zucchini Kabobs

Preparation Time: 8 minutes
Cooking Time: 10 minutes
Serving: 2

Ingredient
- 8 oz extra firm tofu
- 1 medium zucchini, cut into 2-inch rounds
- 1 tbsp olive oil
- 2 tbsp freshly squeezed lemon juice
- 1 tsp smoked paprika
- 1 tsp cumin powder
- ½ tsp parsley dried
- 1 tsp garlic powder

Directions
1. Preheat a grill to medium heat.
2. Meanwhile, thread the tofu and zucchini alternately on the wooden skewers.
3. Scourge olive oil, lemon juice, paprika, parsley, cumin powder, and garlic powder.
4. Brush the skewers all around with the mixture and place on the grill grate. Cook on both sides for 5 minutes. Serve afterward.

Nutrition: 312 Calories 19g Fat 18g Protein

Nutty Tofu Loaf

Preparation Time: 11 minutes
Cooking Time: 62 minutes
Serving: 4

Ingredients
- 2 tbsp olive oil + extra for brushing
- 2 red onions, finely chopped
- 4 garlic cloves, minced
- 1 lb. firm tofu, pressed and crumbled
- 2 tbsp soy sauce
- ¾ cup chopped walnuts
- ¼ cup buckwheat flakes
- 1 tbsp sesame seeds
- 1 cup chopped green bell peppers
- Salt and black pepper to taste
- 1 tbsp Italian seasoning
- ½ tsp brown sugar
- ½ cup tomato sauce

Directions
1. Prepare oven to 350 F and grease an 8 x 4-inch loaf pan with olive oil.
2. Cook 1 tbsp of olive oil in a small skillet and sauté the onion and garlic until softened and fragrant, 2 minutes. Situate onion mixture into a large bowl and mix with the tofu, soy sauce, walnuts, buckwheat flakes, sesame seeds, bell peppers, salt, black pepper, Italian seasoning, and brown sugar.
3. Spoon the mixture into the loaf pan, press to fit, and spread the tomato sauce on top. Bake the tofu loaf in the oven for 45 minutes.
4. Remove the loaf pan from the oven, invert the tofu loaf onto a chopping board, and cool for 5 minutes. Slice and serve warm.

Nutrition: 544 Calories 39g Fat 25g Protein

Chili Toasted Nuts

Preparation Time: 12 minutes
Cooking Time: 33 minutes
Serving: 4

Ingredients
- 1 cup walnuts nuts
- 1 tbsp extra-virgin olive oil, melted
- ¼ tsp hot sauce
- ¼ tsp garlic powder
- ¼ tsp onion powder

Directions
1. Set oven at 350 F and line a baking sheet with baking paper.
2. In a medium bowl, mix the nuts, olive oil, hot sauce, garlic powder, and onion powder. Lay mixture on the baking sheet and toast in the oven for 10 minutes.
3. Remove the sheet, allow complete cooling, and serve.

Nutrition: 267 Calories 25g Fat 6g Protein

Creole Tofu Scramble with Kale

Preparation Time: 9 minutes
Cooking Time: 42 minutes
Serving: 2

Ingredients
- 2 tbsp extra-virgin olive oil, for frying
- 1 (14 oz) pack firm tofu, pressed and crumbled
- 4 green chilies, deseeded and chopped

- 1 tomato, finely chopped
- 2 tbsp chopped fresh green onions
- Salt and black pepper to taste
- 1 tsp turmeric powder
- 1 tsp Creole seasoning
- ½ cup chopped baby kale
- ¼ cup grated Parmesan cheese

Direction
1. Preheat olive oil in a huge skillet over medium heat and cook the tofu with occasional stirring until light golden brown. Make sure not to break the tofu into tiny bits but to have scrambled egg resemblance, 5 minutes.
2. Stir in the chilies, tomato, green onions, salt, black pepper, turmeric powder, and Creole seasoning. Sauté until the vegetables soften, 5 minutes.
3. Mix in the kale to wilt, 3 minutes, and then half of Parmesan cheese. Melt for 2 minutes and turn the heat off. Dish the food, top with the remaining cheese, and serve warm.

Nutrition: 258 Calories 16g Fat 21g Protein

Vegetable Frittata with Red Onions & Green Chilies

Preparation Time: 13 minutes
Cooking Time: 27 minutes
Serving: 1

Ingredients
- 1 tbsp extra-virgin olive oil
- ½ small red onion, chopped
- 1 green chili pepper, chopped
- ½ carrot, chopped
- ½ zucchini, chopped
- 1 tsp turmeric
- 3 eggs
- Salt and black pepper to taste
- 1 tbsp fresh parsley, chopped

Directions
1. Preheat the oven to 350°F.
2. Warmup olive oil in a pan over medium heat. Stir in red onions and sauté for 3 minutes until tender. Pour in carrot, zucchini, and green chili, and cook for 4 minutes. Remove the mixture to a greased baking pan with cooking spray.
3. In a bowl, whisk the eggs with turmeric, salt, and pepper and pour over vegetables. Bake for 10-15 minutes until golden. Drizzle with freshly chopped parsley and serve.

Nutrition: 288 Calories 23g Fat 13g Protein

Sirtfood Frittata

Preparation Time: 8 minutes
Cooking Time: 16 minutes
Serving: 2

Ingredients
- 2 tsp olive oil
- 1 small red onion, chopped
- 2 garlic cloves, chopped
- 4 eggs, beaten
- 2 tomatoes, sliced
- 1 green chili, minced
- 2 tbsp fresh parsley, chopped
- Salt and black pepper, to taste

Directions
1. Set a pan over high heat and warm the olive oil. Sauté garlic and red onion until tender.
2. Whisk the eggs with yogurt. Pour into the pan and cook until eggs become puffy and brown to bottom. Add parsley, chili pepper and tomatoes to one side of the omelet. Season with black pepper and salt. Fold the omelet in half and slice into wedges.

Nutrition: 319 Calories 25g Fat 14g Protein

Baby Arugula Stuffed Zucchini

Preparation Time: 11 minutes
Cooking Time: 42 minutes
Servings: 2

Ingredients
- 2 zucchinis, halved
- 4 tbsp olive oil
- 2 garlic cloves, minced
- 1½ oz baby arugula
- Salt and black pepper to taste
- 2 tbsp tomato sauce
- 1 cup Parmesan cheese, shredded

Directions
1. Scoop out the pulp of the zucchinis into a plate. Keep the flesh. Grease a baking

sheet with cooking spray and place in the zucchini halves.
2. Preheat olive oil in a skillet at medium heat. Sauté the garlic until fragrant, about 1 minute. Add arugula and zucchini pulp. Cook until the arugula wilts; season with salt and pepper. Spoon the tomato sauce into the boats and spread to coat the bottom.
3. Spoon the arugula mixture into the zucchinis and sprinkle with the vegan parmesan cheese. Bake for 24 minutes at 370°F. Plate the zucchinis when ready, season with salt and black pepper.

Nutrition: 520 Calories 37g Fat 20g Protein

Celery Buckwheat Croquettes

Preparation Time: 9 minutes
Cooking time: 25 minutes
Serving: 2

Ingredients
- ¾ cup buckwheat groats, cooked
- 3 tbsp extra-virgin olive oil
- ¼ cup minced red onion
- 1 celery stalk, chopped
- ¼ cup shredded carrots
- 1/3 cup buckwheat flour
- ¼ cup chopped fresh parsley
- Salt and black pepper to taste

Directions
1. Place the groats in a bowl. Cook 1 tbsp of oil in a skillet over medium heat. Place in onion, celery, and carrot and stir-fry for 5 minutes. Transfer to the buckwheat bowl.
2. Mix in flour, parsley, salt, and pepper. Place in the fridge for 20 minutes. Mold the mixture into cylinder-shaped balls. Warm up remaining oil in a skillet over medium heat. Fry the croquettes for 8 minutes, turning occasionally until golden.

Nutrition: 230 Calories 10g Fat 6g Protein

Creole Tempeh & Black Bean Bowls

Preparation Time: 7 minutes
Cooking Time: 50 minutes
Servings: 4

Ingredients
- 2 tbsp olive oil
- 1 ½ cups crumbled tempeh
- 1 tsp Creole seasoning
- 2 red bell peppers, deseeded and sliced
- 2 cups vegetable broth
- Salt to taste
- 1 (8 oz) can black beans, drained and rinsed
- 2 chives, chopped
- 2 tbsp freshly chopped parsley

Direction
1. Cook olive oil in a medium pot and cook in the tempeh until golden brown, 5 minutes. Season with the Creole seasoning and stir in the bell peppers. Cook until the peppers slightly soften, 3 minutes.
2. Stir in the beans, vegetable broth, and salt. Cover and cook for 10 minutes. Stir in the chives and dish the food, garnished with the parsley.

Nutrition: 216 Calories 18g Fat 21g Protein

Spicy Broccoli Pasta

Preparation Time: 6 minutes
Cooking Time: 24 minutes
Serving: 2

Ingredients
- 5 oz buckwheat fusilli
- 4 oz broccoli florets
- 1 tbsp extra-virgin olive oil
- 1 small red onion, finely sliced
- 1 garlic clove, finely sliced
- ½ tsp crushed chilies
- ½ tsp caraway seeds
- 1 large zucchini, coarsely grated
- 4 tbsp low-fat heavy milk
- ½ lemon, zested and juiced
- 3-4 ice cubes

Directions
1. Prepare the pasta according to package instructions. 4 minutes before the end, add in the broccoli to the pan. Drain and keep 3 tbsp of the pasta water.
2. Preheat oil in a huge skillet over a low heat. Add the onion and cook for 5 mins, then stir in the garlic, crushed chilies and caraway seeds. Cook 4-5 minutes more. Add the zucchini and season to taste. Fry until the zucchini is tender, 2 minutes.

3. Add the pasta, broccoli and reserved pasta water to the skillet. Take out from the heat and stir in the heavy cream and lemon juice. Serve warm.

Nutrition: 304 Calories 10g Fat 11g Protein

Buckwheat Pilaf with Pine Nuts

Preparation Time: 13 minutes
Cooking time: 24 minutes
Serves: 2

Ingredients
- 1 cup buckwheat groats
- 2 cups vegetable stock
- ¼ cup walnuts
- 2 tbsp olive oil
- ½ red onion, chopped
- 1/3 cup chopped fresh parsley

Directions
1. Put the groats and vegetable stock in a pot. Bring to a boil, then lower the heat and simmer for 15 minutes. Heat a skillet over medium heat. Place in the pine nuts and toast for 2-3 minutes, shaking often. Heat the oil in the same skillet and sauté the onion for 3 minutes until translucent.
2. Once the groats are ready, fluff them using a fork. Mix in walnuts, onion, and parsley. Sprinkle with salt and pepper. Serve.

Nutrition: 277 Calories 19g Fat 5g Protein

Buckwheat Savoy Cabbage Rolls with Tofu

Preparation Time: 8 minutes
Cooking Time: 31 minutes
Serving: 2

Ingredients
- 2 tbsp extra-virgin olive oil
- 2 cups extra firm tofu, pressed and crumbled
- ½ medium red onion, finely chopped
- 2 garlic cloves, minced
- Salt and black pepper to taste
- 1 cup buckwheat groats
- 1 ¾ cups vegetable stock
- 1 bay leaf
- 2 tbsp chopped fresh cilantro + more for garnishing
- 1 head Savoy cabbage, leaves separated (scraps kept)
- 1 (23 oz) canned chopped tomatoes

Directions
1. Heat olive oil in a big skillet and cook the tofu until golden brown, 8 minutes. Cook onion and garlic for 3 minutes. Season with salt, black pepper and mix in the buckwheat, bay leaf, and vegetable stock.
2. Close the lid, allow boiling, and then simmer until all the liquid is absorbed. Open the lid; remove the bay leaf, adjust the taste with salt, black pepper, and mix in the cilantro.
3. Spread-out cabbage leaves on a flat surface and add 3 to 4 tablespoons of the cooked buckwheat onto each leaf. Roll the leaves to firmly secure the filling.
4. Pour the tomatoes with juices into a medium pot, season with a little salt, black pepper, and lay the cabbage rolls in the sauce. Cook over medium heat until the cabbage softens, 5 to 8 minutes. Turn the heat off and dish the food onto serving plates. Garnish with more cilantro and serve warm.

Nutrition: 598 Calories 28g Fat 48g Protein

Potato and Chickpea Bake

Preparation Time: 18 minutes
Cooking Time: 42 minutes
Serving: 6

Ingredients:
- 1 large baking potato – pricked
- 1 teaspoon olive oil – extra virgin
- ½ red onion – chopped
- 1 garlic clove – mi9nced
- ½ teaspoon ginger – freshly grated
- Chili flakes to taste
- 1 teaspoon cumin seeds
- 1 teaspoon turmeric
- 1 cup tomatoes – tinned chopped
- ½ teaspoon cocoa powder – unsweetened
- 1 cup chickpeas with water
- 1 yellow pepper – chopped
- 1 tablespoon parsley
- Salt to taste

Directions:

1. Prep the oven to 425 degrees F. Once you place a potato in the oven, you will be baking for an hour or until the potato is ready for your taste. Next, take a frying pan and add the olive oil.
2. Set the heat to low medium and add onions to the pan. Cover with the lid and cook on low heat for 5 minutes. When you remove the lid, add ginger, chili, cumin, and garlic. Cook for a minute then add a splash of water and turmeric.
3. Add tomatoes, cocoa, chickpeas, and yellow pepper. Bring the mixture to a simmer on low medium heat – you will be cooking the mixture between 30 and 40 minutes until the sauce thickens. Add salt to taste and parsley, and top the baked potato with the chickpeas sauce.

Nutrition: 268 Calories 4g Fat 9g Protein

Kale Dhal with Buckwheat

Preparation Time: 8 minutes
Cooking Time: 16 minutes
Serving: 5

Ingredients:
- 1 tablespoon extra-virgin olive oil
- 4 garlic cloves – minced
- 2cm piece ginger – grated
- 1 red onion – chopped
- 1 bird's eye chili – finely sliced
- 2 teaspoons garam masala
- 2 teaspoons turmeric
- 150 grams lentils – red
- 400 ml of coconut milk
- 100 grams kale
- 160 grams buckwheat
- 200 ml of water

Directions:
1. Take a deep skillet or a frying pan and add the oil. Heat up the pan then add the onions. Set on the low medium heat and cover the pan while the onion is cooking on low heat for 5 minutes. Remove the lid and add ginger, chili, and garlic.
2. Cook for another minute. Add masala and turmeric with a splash of water and cook for a minute. Blend coconut milk with 200 ml of water and add it to the pan. Add lentils and stir well to combine all ingredients in the pan then cook for 20 minutes with occasional stirring on low medium heat.
3. Place the lid on while cooking. Check for the dhal consistency and add more water if the mass is thickening. After 20 minutes, open lid and add kale.
4. Stir in to combine kale with the rest of the ingredients and cook on low heat for 5 minutes. 5 minutes after you start cooking the dhal with lentils, take a saucepan and add buckwheat with plenty of water.
5. Cook buckwheat for 10 minutes after bringing the water to a boil or until the buckwheat is soft enough to suit your taste. Serve dhal with buckwheat and enjoy your meal.

Nutrition: 209 Calories 6g Fat 10g Protein

Braised Puy Lentils

Preparation Time: 17 minutes
Cooking Time: 22 minutes
Serving: 6

Ingredients:
- 40 grams carrots – sliced
- 40 grams celery – sliced
- 75 grams Puy lentils
- 220 ml of vegetable stock
- 20 grams rocket salad
- 5 grams kale – chopped
- 1 tablespoon parsley – chopped
- 1 teaspoon thyme
- 1 teaspoon paprika
- 1 garlic clove – chopped
- 10 cherry tomatoes
- 2 tablespoons extra virgin olive oil
- 1 red onion - diced

Directions:
1. Prep the oven to 240 degrees F. Situate tomatoes on a small tin and bake for 35 to 40 minutes. As tomatoes are baking, set the stove on low-medium heat and add 1 tablespoon of olive oil, garlic, onion, celery, and carrots. Cook for 2 minutes with occasional stirring. Add paprika and thyme once the veggies are softened and stir in well to combine.
2. Wash and strain lentils then add them to the pan with the vegetable stock. Bring the

mixture to a simmer. Place the lid on and cook for 20 minutes on low heat.
3. Make sure to check the pan every 6 to 7 minutes and add water if necessary. Add kale and remove the lid.
4. Continue cook for 10 minutes then add parsley and tomatoes. Serve with rocket salad. Add the remaining olive oil to the rocket salad.

Nutrition: 213 Calories 16g Fat 23g Protein

Chicken Chili with Buckwheat

Preparation Time: 14 minutes
Cooking Time: 32 minutes
Serving: 5

Ingredients:
- 1 red onion – chopped
- 3 garlic cloves – chopped
- 2 bird's eye chili peppers – sliced
- 400 grams chicken – minced – you can choose thighs or breasts
- 150 ml red wine
- 1 red pepper – cored, deseeded and chopped
- 150 grams kidney beans – tinned
- 300 ml vegetable or chicken stock
- 400 grams tinned chopped tomatoes
- 1 tablespoon extra-virgin olive oil
- 1 tablespoon turmeric – ground
- 1 tablespoon cumin – ground
- 1 tablespoon tomato puree
- 1 tablespoon cocoa powder
- 5 grams parsley – chopped
- 160 grams buckwheat

Directions:
1. Take a skillet and add oil, set the heat to medium and add garlic, chili, and onion once the oil is heated. Cook for 2 minutes with occasional stirring. Add the spices from the in gradient list and cook for another minute. Stir in to combine then add the minced chicken and cook on high heat until the chicken is lightly browned and mixed with spices and onions.
2. Add the red wine. Cook until the wi9ne is reduced by half. Add kidney beans, tomatoes, puree, red pepper, cocoa, and stock. Simmer for one hour. You may need to add water in the middle of cooking to achieve preferred consistency.
3. After the chili is cooked, add chopped herbs, stir in and serve with buckwheat. Cook the buckwheat according to direction on the package.

Nutrition: 226 Calories 8g Fat 19g Protein

Chickpea and Quinoa Curry

Preparation Time: 18 minutes
Cooking Time: 37 minutes
Serving: 4

Ingredients:
- 500 grams potatoes
- 3 garlic cloves – crushed
- 400 ml can coconut milk
- 400 grams chickpeas – canned
- 300 ml boiled water
- 180 grams quinoa
- 150 grams spinach
- 1 tablespoon tomato puree
- 3 teaspoons turmeric – ground
- 1 teaspoon coriander – ground
- 1 teaspoon ginger - ground
- 1 teaspoon chili flakes
- Salt to taste

Directions:
1. Place quartered potatoes in a pot filled with water, add a pinch of salt and bring the water to a boil. Cook for around 25 minutes after the boiling point until you can easily cut through potatoes with a knife.
2. Drain potatoes once cooked until no water is left. Transfer potatoes to a large pan then add turmeric, garlic, chili, ginger, coconut milk, coriander, tomato puree, and tomatoes and bring it all to boil and add salt. Mix well then add quinoa with 300 ml of boiled water. Set heat to low-medium and let the mixture simmer.
3. Cover the pan and allow the curry to cook for the next 30 minutes. Stir the curry every 5 minutes or so. Make sure that none of the ingredients are sticking to the bottom of the pan. After 15 minutes of cooking, add the chickpeas, stir in and cover the pot again.

4. When you are at the last 5 minutes of cooking, add spinach and stir in. You will know that the curry is ready when quinoa becomes soft instead of crunchy.

Nutrition: 333 Calories 12g Fat 14g Protein

Vegetable Chili

Preparation Time: 16 minutes
Cooking Time: 34 minutes
Serving: 4

Ingredients:
- ½ cup zucchini – fresh, chopped
- 50 grams Cremini mushrooms
- 2 cups tomatoes – diced
- 1 cup kidney beans – canned
- ½ cup red onion – chopped
- 1 tablespoon olive oil
- ½ cup red bell pepper – chopped
- 2 teaspoons cumin seeds – ground
- 1 teaspoon chili powder
- ½ bird's eye chili – sliced
- 1 garlic clove – minced

Directions:
1. Cook tablespoon of olive oil in a skillet over medium-high heat. Add the onions and garlic and sauté while occasionally stirring for a minute or two.
2. Add zucchini, peppers, and mushrooms. Sauté and stir for another 2 minutes or so, then add cumin and chili powder. After combining all the ingredients add the beans and tomatoes.
3. Bring the mixture to a boil. Adjust heat to medium and simmer for the next 20 to 30 minutes. Serve and enjoy.

Nutrition: 157 Calories 2g Fat 7g Protein

Lemon Splash Tofu

Preparation Time: 9 minutes
Cooking Time: 13 minutes
Serving: 3

Ingredients:
- 250 grams firm tofu – extra firm
- ½ teaspoon lemon zest – freshly grated
- ¼ lemon – peeled, fresh
- 1/8 cup sundried tomatoes
- 1 garlic clove
- ½ teaspoon ground fennel seeds
- 1 tablespoon extra-virgin olive oil

Direction:
1. Prepare the oven to 400 degrees F. Combine olive oil, tomatoes, fennel, crushed garlic, and lemon zest to make a marinade for the tofu. Lightly oil a baking dish then cut the tofu into four equal pieces.
2. Coat the top of the pieces with some of the marinade. Arrange the pieces in the baking dish. Bake for 13 minutes. Serve with the rest of the marinade and enjoy your dish.

Nutrition: 254 Calories 20g Fat 14g Protein

Veggie Stuffed Peppers

Preparation Time: 14 minutes
Cooking Time: 36 minutes
Serving: 6

Ingredients:
- 1 green pepper
- ¾ cup brown rice - cooked
- 2 tablespoons red onion – diced
- 2 tablespoons celery – diced
- ¼ cup tomato puree
- ½ bird's eye chili – finely sliced
- ½ teaspoon oregano - dry
- ½ teaspoon basil – dry
- ½ teaspoon thyme – ground
- 2 slices Mozzarella cheese
- 2 tablespoons olive oil

Directions:
1. Preheat skillet with a tablespoon of olive oil on medium heat. Add onions and celery and diced green pepper to the skillet. Sauté for one to two minutes.
2. Add tomato puree then cook for five minutes while simmering. Add the herbs and spices and stir in to combine. Add the brown rice and stir in to combine all the ingredients.
3. Take the whole pepper – top off and deseeded - and cut it in half across the length. Stuff each half with rice mixture. Situate one slice of cheese on each half then place in a lightly greased up baking dish. Bake over 350 degrees F for 23 minutes. Serve and enjoy!

Nutrition: 405 Calories 15g Fat 18g Protein

Veggie Jambalaya

Preparation Time: 12 minutes

Cooking Time: 29 minutes
Serving: 3
Ingredients:
- ¼ cup dark red beans – canned
- ¼ cup red onion – chop
- ¼ cup red bell pepper – chopped
- ¼ cup yellow pepper – chopped
- ¾ cups brown rice - cooked
- 1 garlic clove – minced
- 50 grams tomato paste – canned
- 25 grams silk five-grain tempeh
- ½ cup vegetable broth
- 1 bird's eye chili pepper
- 1 tablespoon extra-virgin olive oil
- Salt to taste

Directions:
1. Prep skillet on medium-high heat and add the oil. Add garlic and onion and sauté for a minute or two.
2. Reduce the heat to medium. Add sliced tempeh and peppers and cook until the veggies are softened to your preference. Add the spices and salt, broth, and tomato paste. Stir in to combine then bring the mixture to a simmer.
3. Once the jambalaya starts to simmer, add cooked brown rice and stir to combine. Serve while hot and enjoy your lunch.

Nutrition: 509 Calories 16g Fat 15g Protein

Veggie Stir Fry

Preparation Time: 9 minutes
Cooking Time: 24 minutes
Serving: 4
Ingredients:
- ¼ cup red onion – chopped
- ¼ cup broccoli – florets, chopped
- ¼ cup mushrooms – chopped
- ¼ cup red sweet pepper – chopped
- 1 bird's eye chili – sliced
- 1 tablespoon extra-virgin olive oil
- Salt to taste
- 1 tablespoon dark soy sauce

Directions:
1. Ready skillet on medium heat and add a tablespoon of oil. Once the oil is heated, add the veggies, sprinkling salt afterward.
2. Coat the veggies and cook the veggies. Add a tablespoon of soy sauce at the end, stir and serve hot.

Nutrition: 180 Calories 14g Fat 2g Protein

Buckwheat Pasta Salad

Preparation Time: 8 minutes
Cooking Time: 26 minutes
Serving: 2
Ingredients:
- 50 grams buckwheat pasta
- 50 grams rocket salad
- ½ avocado – peeled and diced
- 10 cherry tomatoes
- 10 olives
- 1 tablespoon extra-virgin olive oil
- 20 grams pine nuts

Directions:
1. Cook the buckwheat pasta as per to the instructions on the package. As the pasta is cooking, you will prepare the rest of the ingredients.
2. Drain the pasta and rinse it under the cold water. Combine all ingredients except the pine nuts. Top the salad with pine nuts.

Nutrition: 220 Calories 3g Fat 7g Protein

Greek Salad on a Stick

Preparation Time: 21 minutes
Cooking Time: 0 minute
Serving: 1
Ingredients:
- 2 skewers – wooden
- 8 black olives
- 1 red pepper – cut in 8 pieces
- 1 yellow pepper – cut in 8 pieces
- 100 grams cucumber – cut into cubes
- 100 grams feta cheese – cut into 8 pieces
- ½ red onion – cut into 8 pieces

Dressing:
- 1 tablespoon extra-virgin olive oil
- ½ lemon – juiced
- 1 teaspoon vinegar – balsamic
- 1 garlic clove – crushed
- Several leaves of basil - fresh
- Several leaves of oregano – fresh
- Salt to taste

Directions:

1. Submerge wooden skewers in warm water for 30 minutes before threading the ingredients. Prepare the Greek salad on skewers by threading all ingredients, previously preparing all the veggies and cheese for threading.
2. Thread the ingredients first threading olives, cherry tomatoes, cucumber, pepper, and feta cheese – repeat the process by threading ingredients in the same order.
3. Prepare the dressing by placing all ingredients from the dressing list in a bowl. Mix all ingredients then pour over the Greek salad on skewers.

Nutrition: 306 Calories 1g Fat 5g Protein

Tofu Curry

Preparation Time: 18 minutes
Cooking Time: 31 minutes
Serving: 5

Ingredients:
- 1-liter water
- 1 tablespoon grapeseed oil
- 1 red onion – chopped
- 1 bird's eye chili
- 4 garlic cloves – chopped
- 1 teaspoon paprika
- ¼ teaspoon cayenne pepper
- ½ teaspoon turmeric – ground
- 7cm piece of ginger – grated
- 1 teaspoon salt
- 250 grams red lentils – dry
- 50 grams edamame beans – frozen
- 200 grams tofu – firm, cubed
- 1 lime - juiced
- 200 grams kale
- 2 tomatoes - chopped

Directions:
1. Put stove to low medium heat and put the oil in a pan. Add onions and cook for 5 minutes with occasional stirring. After the onions are cooked, add ginger, garlic, and chili.
2. Cook for 2 more minutes then add cumin, salt, cayenne, paprika, and turmeric. Stir the ingredients to combine with the onion mixture then add the lentils. As you are preparing this base for your dish, take a large cooking pot and pour 1 liter of water.
3. Boil water then add the boiling water to the pan to bring the ingredients to simmer for 10 minutes. Set heat to low and allow the curry to cook for 20 to 30 minutes on low heat and until the consistency of the dish is porridge-like.
4. Add edamame beans, tofu, and tomatoes. Cook the curry for another 5 minutes after adding the three ingredients then add lime juice and kale. Cook until kale is softened. Serve warm and enjoy.

Nutrition: 342 Calories 5g Fat 28g Protein

Veggie and Buckwheat Stir

Preparation Time: 7 minutes
Cooking Time: 32 minutes
Serving: 4

Ingredients:
- ½ cup buckwheat
- 3 tablespoons extra virgin olive oil
- 1 cup of water
- 1 medium carrot
- 1 medium red onion
- 1 red bell pepper -diced, deseeded
- 1 yellow bell pepper – diced, deseeded
- 10 grams parsley - chopped

Directions:
1. Take a heavy bottom pan and add buckwheat. Cook for 5 minutes on medium-low with frequent stirring and with no oil or water. Buckwheat can easily burn, so make sure to stir while cooking for the first 5 minutes.
2. Cook 1 tablespoon of oil and stir in well. Mix and stir frequently until the oil is absorbed then add a cup of water.
3. Set heat to low, bring to a simmer, and cover with a lid. Cook for 20 minutes on low. Once you remove buckwheat from the heat don't open the lid but let it sit for another 20 minutes.
4. Pre-heat two tablespoons of oil in a skillet then add the onions, carrots, and peppers. Add some salt then stir to combine. Cook the veggies until softened.
5. Remove the lid from buckwheat then stir and add a sprinkle of salt. Add the sautéed veggies then stir to combine. Add parsley as a garnish and enjoy your meal.

Nutrition: 198 Calories 5g Fat 6g Protein

Sweet Pepper Mix

Preparation Time: 14 minutes
Cooking Time: 0 minute
Serving: 3

Ingredients:
- 1/8 cup green bell pepper
- ¼ cup red bell pepper
- 1/8 cup yellow pepper
- 1/8 cup red onion
- ¼ cup rocket salad
- 1 tablespoon parsley – chopped
- ¼ lemon - juiced

Directions:
1. Dice the bell peppers, onion, and parsley and combine with rocket salad. Mix to combine in a salad bowl then dress with lemon juice.

Nutrition: 34 Calories 0.1g Fat 0.5g Protein

Cottage Cheese Veggie Salad

Preparation Time: 14 minutes
Cooking Time: 0 minute
Servings: 2

Ingredients:
- 6 cherry tomatoes
- ½ cup cottage cheese
- 2 tbsps. scallion
- 2 green olives

Directions:
1. Slice five tomatoes into quarters; set aside remaining tomato for garnish.
2. Mix all ingredients except lettuce and garnish
3. Garnish with cheese mixture, and reserved cherry tomato.

Nutrition: 342 Calories 27g Fat 12g Protein

Arugula and Lemon Rice

Preparation Time: 7 minutes
Cooking Time: 37 minutes
Servings: 5

Ingredients:
- 1 red onion
- 1 cup mushrooms
- 2 cloves garlic
- 1 tbsp. olive oil
- 3 cup long-grain rice
- 10 oz. arugula
- 3 tbsp. lemon juice
- ¼ tsp. dill weed
- 1/3 cup feta cheese

Directions:
1. Set oven at 350°F. Cook onion, mushrooms and garlic in oil. Mix in the rice, arugula, lemon juice, dill and season well.
2. Set aside 1 tbsp. cheese and mix rest into skillet. Situate to greased 8-in. square baking dish. Drizzle with reserved cheese. Bake for 25 minutes.
3. Uncover then bake until heated through and cheese is melted.

Nutrition: 367 Calories 21g Fat 17g Protein

Spring Pesto Beans

Preparation time: 9 minutes
Cooking Time: 60 minutes
Servings: 3

Ingredients:
- 2 tbsp. Olive oil
- 2 tsp. Sweet paprika
- 1 lemon juice
- 2 tbsp. Basil pesto
- 1 lb. green beans
- ¼ tsp. black pepper
- 1 red onion

Direction:
1. Preheat pan with the oil at medium-high heat; cook onion for 5 minutes.
2. Cook beans and the rest of the ingredients for 11 minutes, then serve.

Nutrition: 312 Calories 26g Fat 8g Protein

Mung Sprouts Salsa

Preparation Time: 9 minutes
Cooking Time: 0 minute
Servings: 2

Ingredients:
- 1 red onion, chopped
- 2 c. mung beans, sprouted
- A pinch of red chili powder
- 1 green chili pepper, chopped
- 1 tomato, chopped
- 1 tsp. Chaat masala
- 1 tsp. lemon juice
- 1 tbsp. coriander, chopped
- Black pepper to the taste

Directions:
1. In a salad bowl, mix onion with mung sprouts, chili pepper, tomato, chili powder, Chaat masala, lemon juice, coriander and pepper, toss well, divide into small cups and serve.

Nutrition: 321 Calories 19g Fat 7g Protein

Honey Chili Squash

Preparation Time: 16 minutes
Cooking Time: 33 minutes
Servings: 2

Ingredients:
- 2 red onions, roughly chopped 2.5cm
- 1-inch chunk of ginger root, finely chopped
- 2 cloves garlic
- 2 bird's-eye chilies, finely chopped
- 1 butternut squash, peeled and chopped
- 100 ml (3½ fl. oz.) vegetable stock broth
- 1 tbsp. olive oil
- Juice of 1 orange
- Juice of 1 lime
- 2 tsps. honey

Directions:
1. Warm the oil into a pan and add in the red onions, squash chunks, chilies, garlic, ginger and honey. Cook for 3 minutes.
2. Squeeze in the lime and orange juice. Pour in the stock broth), orange and lime juice and cook for 15 minutes until tender.

Nutrition: 300 Calories 14g Fat 6g Protein

Salsa Bean Dip

Preparation Time: 9 minutes
Cooking Time: 22 minutes
Servings: 6

Ingredients:
- ½ c. salsa
- 2 c. canned white beans, no-salt-added, drained and rinsed
- 1 c. low-fat cheddar, shredded
- 2 tbsps. green onions, chopped

Directions:
1. Simmer beans with the green onions and salsa over medium heat for 20 minutes.
2. Mix cheese, until it melts, put off heat, set aside then serve.

Nutrition: 271 Calories 20g Fat 7g Protein

Roast Balsamic Vegetables

Preparation Time: 7 minutes
Cooking Time: 44 minutes
Servings: 2

Ingredients:
- 4 tomatoes, chopped
- 2 red onions, chopped
- 3 sweet potatoes, peeled and chopped
- 100g (3½ oz.) red chicory or if unavailable, use yellow
- 100g (3½ oz.) kale, finely chopped
- 300g (11 oz.) potatoes, peeled and chopped
- 5 stalks celery, chopped
- 1 bird's-eye chili, de-seeded and finely chopped
- 2 tbsps. fresh parsley, chopped
- 2 tbsps. fresh coriander cilantro chopped
- 3 tbsps. olive oil
- 2 tbsps. balsamic vinegar 1 teaspoon mustard
- Sea salt
- Freshly ground black pepper

Directions:
1. Place the olive oil, balsamic, mustard, parsley and coriander cilantro into a bowl and mix well.
2. Toss all the remaining ingredients into the dressing and season with salt and pepper. Transfer the vegetables to an ovenproof dish and cook in the oven at 200C/400F for 45 minutes.

Nutrition: 299 Calories 19g Fat 4g Protein

Courgette and Tomato Risotto

Preparation Time: 8 minutes
Cooking Time: 17 minutes
Servings: 9

Ingredients:
- 2 tbsp. olive oil
- 4 garlic cloves
- 1 ½ lb. Rice Arborio
- 6 tomatoes
- 2 tsp. chop rosemary
- 6 courgette
- 1 ¼ cup peas
- 12 cup hot vegetable stock

Directions:

1. Situate big, heavy-bottomed pan over medium heat then pour oil.
2. Once heated, sauté onion.
3. Cook the tomatoes then stir in the rice and rosemary. Cook half the stock
4. Cook remaining stock for 3 minutes.
5. Cook courgette and peas.
6. Season well.
7. Mix in the basil and set aside for 5 minutes.

Nutrition: 293 Calories 16g Fat 5g Protein

Black Bean Salsa

Preparation Time: 12 minutes
Cooking Time: 0 minute
Servings: 6

Ingredients:
- 1 tbsp. coconut aminos
- ½ tsp. cumin, ground
- 1 c. canned black beans, no-salt-added, drained and rinsed
- 1 c. salsa
- 6 c. romaine lettuce leaves, torn
- ½ c. avocado, peeled, pitted and cubed

Directions:
1. In a bowl, combine the beans with the aminos, cumin, salsa, lettuce and avocado, toss, divide into small bowls and serve as a snack.

Nutrition: 180 Calories 17g Fat 5g Protein

Brown Basmati Rice Pilaf

Preparation Time: 18 minutes
Cooking Time: 14 minutes
Servings: 2

Ingredients:
- ½ tbsp. vegan butter
- ½ c. mushrooms, chopped
- ½ c. brown basmati rice
- 3 tbsps. water
- 1/8 tsp. dried thyme
- Ground pepper to taste
- ½ tbsp. olive oil
- ¼ c. green onion, chopped
- 1 c. vegetable broth
- ¼ tsp. salt
- ¼ c. chopped, toasted pecans

Directions:
1. Place a saucepan over medium-low heat. Add butter and oil.
2. When it melts, add mushrooms and cook until slightly tender.
3. Stir in the green onion and brown rice. Cook for 3 minutes. Stir constantly.
4. Stir in the broth, water, salt and thyme.
5. When about to boil, reduce heat and cover with a lid. Simmer until rice is cooked.
6. Stir in the pecans and pepper.

Nutrition: 281 Calories 17g Fat 4g Protein

Crunchy Arugula with Apples

Preparation Time: 18 minutes
Cooking Time: 8 minutes
Servings: 3

Ingredients:
- 2 tbsp. olive oil
- 2 garlic cloves
- 2 tbsp. pine nuts
- 1 apple
- 10 ounces arugula

Directions:
1. Preheat olive oil in wok over low heat.
2. Cook the pine nuts, garlic and apple for 4 minutes
3. Adjust heat to medium and cook arugula for 4 minutes. Season it well.

Nutrition: 315 Calories 21g Fat 7g Protein

Cauliflower and Carrots Dip

Preparation Time: 17 minutes
Cooking Time: 32 minutes
Servings: 3

Ingredients:
- 1 cup carrots
- 2 cups cauliflower florets
- ½ cup cashews
- 2 ½ cup water
- 1 cup almond milk
- 1 tsp. garlic powder
- ¼ tsp. paprika

Direction:
1. Boil carrots with cauliflower, cashews and water at medium heat for 40 minutes, strain and place in the blender.
2. Blend almond milk, garlic powder and paprika, then serve

Nutrition: 289 Calories 21g Fat 8g Protein

Kale and Bean Casserole

Preparation Time: 7 minutes

Cooking time: 46 minutes
Servings: 3
Ingredients:
- 1 ½ cup milk
- 1 cup sour cream
- 1 cup mushrooms
- 2 cup green beans
- 2 cup kale
- ¼ cup capers
- ¼ cup walnuts

Direction:
1. Prepare oven to 375 degrees F then grease a casserole dish.
2. Scourge milk and sour cream.
3. Mix in mushrooms, green beans, kale, and capers. Fill into the casserole dish
4. Drizzle with the crushed walnuts.
5. Bake uncovered for 40 minutes.

Nutrition: 308 Calories 24g Fat 8g Protein

Red Coleslaw

Preparation Time: 11 minutes
Cooking Time: 0 minute
Servings: 4
Ingredients:
- 1 2/3 lbs. red cabbage
- 2 tbsps. ground caraway seeds
- 1 tbsp. whole grain mustard
- 1 1/4 c. mayonnaise, low fat, low sodium
- Salt and black pepper

Directions:
1. Cut the red cabbage into small slices.
2. Incorporate all the ingredients alongside cabbage.
3. Mix well, season with salt and pepper.
4. Serve!

Nutrition: 281 Calories 17g Fat 7g Protein

Balsamic Eggplant Salsa

Preparation Time: 18 minutes
Cooking Time: 9 minutes
Servings: 3
Ingredients:
- 1 ½ cup tomatoes
- 3 cup eggplant
- 2 tsp. capers
- 6 oz. green olives
- 4 garlic cloves
- 2 tsp. balsamic vinegar
- 1 tbsp. basil

Direction:
1. Pre-heat pan with the oil over medium-high heat, cook eggplant for 5 minutes.
2. Cook tomatoes, capers, olives, garlic, vinegar, basil and black pepper for 7 minutes then serve cold.

Nutrition: 284 Calories 18g Fat 11g Protein

SEAFOOD RECIPES

Stir-Fried Prawn Noodles

Preparation Time: 19 minutes
Cooking Time: 22 minutes
Serving: 1

Ingredients:
- 5 ounce shelled raw king prawns, deveined
- 2 tsp tamari
- 2 tsp extra virgin olive oil
- soba (buckwheat noodles)
- 1 garlic clove, finely chopped
- 1 bird's eye chili, finely chopped
- 1 tsp finely chopped fresh ginger
- 1-ounce red onions, sliced
- 2-ounce celery, trimmed and sliced
- 3-ounce green beans, chopped
- 2-ounce kale, roughly chopped
- 100ml chicken stock
- 1-ounce lovage or celery leaves

Direction:
1. Warm-up frying pan over a high heat, then cook the prawns for 2–3 minutes in 1 teaspoon tamari and 1 teaspoon oil. Put the prawns onto a plate. Wipe the pan out with paper from the oven, because you would be using it again.
2. Cook the noodles 5–8 minutes in boiling water, or as directed on the packet. Drain and throw aside.
3. While, over medium-high heat, fry the garlic, chili and ginger, red onion, celery, beans and kale in the remaining oil for 2–3 minutes. Attach the stock and bring to the boil, then simmer for one to two minutes until the vegetables are cooked but crunchy.
4. Attach the prawns, noodles and leaves of lovage / celery to the oven, put back to the simmer, then reduce the heat and drink.

Nutrition: 317 Calories 24g Fat 9g Protein

Buckwheat Noodles and Shrimp

Preparation Time: 28 minutes
Cooking Time: 17 minutes
Serving: 1

Ingredients:
- 1/3-pound shelled whole jumbo shrimp, deveined tamari 2 teaspoons
- 2 Extra virgin olive oil Teaspoons
- 3 ounces soba
- 2 Nicely sliced garlic cloves
- 1 Finely minced Thai chili
- 1 tablespoon of beautifully minced fresh ginger
- 1/8 cup red onions
- 1/2 cup sliced celery including leaves
- 1/2 cup green beans, minced
- 3/4 cup kale, roughly chopped
- 1/2 cup chicken stock.

Direction
1. Heat a frying pan over high pressure, then cook the shrimp for 2 minutes in 1 teaspoon tamari and 1 teaspoon oil. Place the shrimp into a tray.
2. Cook the noodles for 7 minutes in boiling water. Drain and throw aside.
3. While, in the remaining tamari and oil over medium-high heat, fry the garlic, chili, ginger, red onion, celery, green beans, and kale for 2 min. Boil stock then simmer for a minute.
4. Attach the shrimp, pasta, and leaves of celery to the plate, bring back to a simmer, then remove and serve from fire.

Nutrition: 417 Calories 28g Fat 13g Protein

Prawn Arrabbiata

Preparation Time: 7 minutes
Cooking Time: 19 minutes
Serving: 1

Ingredients:
- 125-150 g Raw prawns
- 65 g Buckwheat pasta
- 1 tbsp Extra virgin olive oil

For arrabbiata sauce:
- 2-ounce Red onion, finely chopped
- 1 Garlic clove, finely chopped
- 2-ounce Celery, finely chopped
- 1 Bird's eye chili, finely chopped
- 1 tsp Dried mixed herbs
- 1 tsp Extra virgin olive oil
- 2 tbsp White wine (optional)

- 15-ounce Tinned chopped tomatoes
- 1 tbsp Chopped parsley

Direction:
1. Fry the onion, garlic, celery and chili over medium-low heat and dry herbs in the oil for 1–2 minutes. Set to medium heat then add the wine and cook 1 minute. Add the tomatoes and allow the sauce to steam for 20-30 minutes over medium-low heat
2. While cooking the sauce, bring a bowl of water to the boil and cook the pasta according to the Preparation packet. Once cooked, drain, toss with the olive oil and keep aside
3. Add the raw prawns to the sauce and cook for another 4 minutes then add the parsley and serve.
4. Mix in cooked pasta to the sauce and mix well but gently and serve.

Nutrition: 348 Calories 27g Fat 11g Protein

Salmon with Turmeric

Preparation Time: 19 minutes
Cooking Time: 27 minutes
Serving: 1
Ingredients:
- 10-ounce Skinned Salmon
- 1 tsp Extra virgin olive oil
- 1 tsp Ground turmeric
- 1/4 Juice of a lemon
- For the spicy celery
- 1 tsp Extra virgin olive oil
- 2-ounce Red onion, finely chopped
- 3-ounce Tinned green lentils
- 1 Garlic clove, finely chopped
- 1 cm Fresh ginger, finely chopped
- 1 Bier's eye chili, finely chopped
- 150 g Celery, cut into 2cm lengths
- 1 tsp Mild curry powder
- 6-ounce Tomato, cut into 8 wedges
- 100 ml Chicken or vegetable stock
- 1 tbsp Chopped parsley

Direction
1. Heat the oven to 200 C
2. Begin with the spicy celery. Heat over medium-low heat a frying pan, add olive oil, then onion, garlic, ginger, chili and celery. Cook gently for 2minutes, then apply the curry powder and cook about a minute more.
3. Then introduce the tomatoes, stock and lentils and gently simmer for 10 minutes. Depending about how crunchy you want your celery you may want to increasing or decrease the cooking period.
4. In the meanwhile, bring together the turmeric, oil and lemon juice and spray over the salmon. Put on a baking tray and cook 8–10 minutes.
5. Stir the parsley through the celery to end, and serve with salmon.

Nutrition: 411 Calories 31g Fat 20g Protein

Salmon Fillet Pan-Fried

Preparation Time: 9 minutes
Cooking Time: 28 minutes
Serving: 1
Ingredients:
- 1/4 cup lemon parsley juice
- 1 Tbsp. capers
- 1 Clove of garlic, peeled roughly
- 1 tablespoon of extra virgin olive oil
- 1/4 avocado, peeled, stoned, and diced
- 2/3 cup cherry tomatoes, half
- 1/8 cup red onion, thinly sliced
- 13/4 ounces arugula
- 2 tablespoons celery leaves
- 1 x 5-ounce fillet of skinless salmon
- 2 Spoonful of brown sugar
- 1 Endive arm, roughly 21/2 ounces (70 g), halved in length

Direction:
1. Set oven to 220 ° C (425° F).
2. Situate parsley, lemon juice, capers, garlic, and 2 teaspoons of oil in a food processor or mixer for dressing and blend until smooth.
3. For the salad, combine the leaves of avocado, tomato, red onion, arugula, and celery.
4. Heat a fried casserole over high pressure. Roll the salmon in a little oil and sear for a minute or two in the hot pan to caramelize the fish's underside.
5. Switch to a baking tray and put in the oven for 5 to 6 minutes or until it is cooked;

decrease the cooking period by 2 minutes if you want the pink eaten inside of your cod.
6. Wipe the frying pan out meanwhile and put it back on high fire. Blend the brown sugar with the remaining oil tablespoon and pour it over the endive cut sides.
7. Put the cut-sides of the endive in the hot pan and cook for 2 to 3 minutes. In the sauce, mix the salad and eat with tuna, and endive.

Nutrition: 341Calories 29g Fat 13g Protein

Sirt Food Miso Marinated Cod

Preparation Time: 21 minutes
Cooking Time: 17 minutes
Serving: 1

Ingredients:
- 1-ounce miso
- 1 tbsp mirin
- 1 tbsp extra virgin olive oil
- 7-ounce skinless cod fillet
- 1-ounce red onion, sliced
- 2-ounce celery, sliced
- 1 garlic clove, finely chopped
- 1 bird's eye chili, finely chopped
- 1 tsp finely chopped fresh ginger
- 3-ounce green beans
- 3-ounce kale, roughly chopped
- 1 tsp sesame seeds
- 1-ounce parsley, roughly chopped
- 1 tbsp tamari
- 2-ounce buckwheat
- 1 tsp ground turmeric

Direction
1. Incorporate miso, mirin and 1 teaspoon of the oil. Rub all over the cod and marinate for 30 minutes. Heat the oven to a temperature of 220C.
2. Bake the cod for about 10 minutes.
3. Preheat wok with the remaining oil. Sauté onion then add the celery, garlic, chili, ginger, green beans and kale.
4. Cook the buckwheat according to the package instruction: with the turmeric for 3 minutes.
5. Add the sesame seed, the parsley and the tamari to the stir-fry and serve with the greens and the fish.

Nutrition: 407 Calories 21g Fat 13g Protein

Smoked Salmon Omelet

Preparation Time: 19 minutes
Cooking Time: 11 minutes
Serving: 1

Ingredients:
- 2 Medium eggs
- 100 g Smoked salmon, sliced
- 1/2 tsp Capers
- 10 g Rocket, chopped
- 1 tsp Parsley, chopped
- 1 tsp Extra virgin olive oil

Direction:
1. Beat eggs. Add the salmon, the capers, the rocket and the Persil.
2. Pre-heat olive oil in a non-stick frying pan. Pour egg mixture and spread around the pan evenly.
3. Reduce heat and let the omelet cook. Slide the spatula along the sides and roll up or split the omelet in half to eat.

Nutrition: 499 Calories 34g Fat 14g Protein

Seafood Salad

Preparation Time: 22 minutes
Cooking Time: 0 minute
Serving: 1

Ingredients:
- 3-ounce rocket
- 3-ounce chicory leaves
- 4-ounce smoked salmon slices
- 4-ounce avocado, peeled, stoned and sliced
- 2-ounce celery, sliced
- 1-ounce red onion, sliced
- 11-ounce walnuts, chopped
- 1 tbs capers
- 1 large Medjool date, pitted and chopped
- 1 tbs extra-virgin olive oil
- Juice ¼ lemon
- 1-ounce parsley, chopped
- 1-ounce lovage or celery leaves, chopped

Direction
1. Prepare the salad leaves in a plate. Incorporate all the remaining ingredients together and situate on top of the leaves.

Nutrition: 351 Calories 23g Fat 7g Protein

Salmon Pasta Smoked with Chili/Arugula

Preparation Time: 17 minutes
Cooking Time: 26 minutes
Serving: 4

Ingredients:
- 2 Spoonful of extra virgin olive oil
- 1 Orange, finely diced onion
- 2 Teaspoons of garlic, finely minced
- 2 Thai, finely minced chilies
- 1 cup cherry tomatoes
- 1/2 cup (100ml) white wine with half
- Buckwheat pasta: 9 to 11 ounces
- 9 Ounces Smoked Salmon
- 2 Teaspoons capers
- 1/2 lemon juice
- 2 ounces of arugula
- 1/4 cup of minced parsley

Direction
1. In a frying pan flame 1 tablespoon of the oil over medium heat. Stir in the cabbage, garlic, chili and cook until smooth but not dark.
2. Attach the tomatoes and require to cook for one or two minutes. To rising by half, add the white wine and bubble.
3. Boil pasta with 1 tablespoon of oil and water for 9 minutes, then rinse.
4. Break the salmon into pieces and add the capers, lemon juice, arugula and parsley to the tomato saucepan. Attach the sauce, blend together and eat right away. Drizzle some oil left on hand.

Nutrition: 427 Calories 28g Fat 14g Protein

Minty Salmon Salad

Preparation Time: 13 minutes
Cooking time: 19 minutes
Serving: 1

Ingredients:
- 1 salmon fillet (12 ounce)
- 2-ounce mixed salad leaves
- 2-ounce young spinach leaves
- 2 radishes, trimmed and thinly sliced
- 5cm piece cucumber, cut into chunks
- 2 spring onions, trimmed and sliced
- 1 small handful parsley, roughly chopped

For the dressing:
- 1 tsp low-fat mayonnaise
- 1 tbsp natural yogurt
- 1 tbsp rice vinegar
- 2 leaves mint, finely chopped
- Salt and freshly ground black pepper

Direction
1. Pre - heat to 200 ° C (180 ° C fan / Gas 6).
2. Situate salmon filet on a baking tray and bake through for 17 minutes. Take out from the oven.
3. Mix the mayonnaise, mustard, rice wine vinegar, mint leaves then season and leave to stand for at least 5 minutes to allow the aromas to form.
4. Arrange the salad leaves and spinach with cucumber, radishes, spring onions and parsley.
5. Put cooked salmon over the salad and sprinkle over the dressing.

Nutrition: 328 Calories 27g Fat 13g Protein

Stir-Fry Shrimp and Buckwheat

Preparation Time: 18 minutes
Cooking Time: 24 minutes
Serving: 1

Ingredients
- Shelled raw jumbo shrimp, deveined 1/3 pound (150g)
- Tamari 2 teaspoons
- Extra virgin olive oil 2 teaspoons
- Soba (buckwheat noodles) 3 ounces (75g)
- Garlic cloves, finely sliced 2
- Thai chili, finely sliced 1
- Teaspoon finely sliced fresh ginger 1
- Red onions, sliced 1/8 cup (20g)
- Celery 1/2 cup (45g)
- Green beans, chopped 1/2 cup (75g)
- Kale, roughly chopped 3/4 cup (50g)
- Chicken stock 1/2 cup

Direction
1. Steam a deep fryer over high temperature, then cook the shrimp for two or three minutes in 1 tablespoon tamari and one teaspoon oil. Put the shrimp into a tray. Flush the skillet out with a towel of paper, as you will be using it again.

2. Bake the noodles for five to eight minutes in boiling water, or as indicated on the box. Flush and put away.
3. Elsewhere, in the leftover tamari and oil over medium-high heat, cook the garlic, ginger, chili, celery, red onion, (but not the leaves), kale and green beans for two to three min. Remove the stocks and bring to a simmer, then steam for a couple of minutes until baked and yet crunchy.
4. Add the shrimp, pasta, and foliage of celery to the bowl, bring to a simmer, turn off the heat and drink.

Nutrition: 417 Calories 28g Fat 13g Protein

Pan-Fried Salmon Fillet with Leafy Salad

Preparation Time: 14 minutes
Cooking time: 19 minutes
Serving: 1

Ingredients
- Parsley 1/4 cup
- Juice of lemon ¼
- Capers 1 tablespoon
- Clove garlic, roughly chopped 1
- Extra-virgin olive oil 1 tablespoon
- Avocado 1/4
- Cherry tomatoes, 2/3 cup
- Red onion, thinly sliced 1/8 cup
- Arugula 1 3/4 ounces
- Celery leaves 2 tablespoons
- Skinless salmon fillet 1 x 5-ounce
- Brown sugar 2 teaspoons
- Head of endive 1

Direction
1. Heat the oven up to 220 ° C (425oF).
2. Put the parsley, garlic, lemon juice, capers, and two teaspoons of oil in a mixing bowl or blender for dressing and mix until thick and creamy.
3. For the salad, combine the leaves of red onion, tomato, arugula, avocado and celery.
4. Warm a frying casserole over high temperature. Massage the salmon in a little oil and sear for a moment or so in the frying skillet to caramelize the exterior. Exchange to a small bowl and bake in the oven for four to six minutes or until it is finished cooking; decrease the heating process by two minutes if you like the pink presented inside of your fish.
5. Wash the saucepan out afterwards and put everything back on high fire. Mix the brown sugar with the remaining oil teaspoon and sprinkle it over the endive cut sides.
6. Position the sides of the endive cut into the skillet and cook for two or three minutes, trying to turn frequently, until tender and perfectly golden brown. In the sauce, mix the salad and top with tuna, and endive.

Nutrition: 371 Calories 28g Fat 7g Protein

Miso-Marinated Baked Cod

Preparation time: 17 minutes
Cooking Time: 29 minutes
Serving: 1

Ingredients
- Miso 3 1/2 teaspoons
- Mirin 1 tablespoon
- Extra-virgin olive oil 1 tablespoon
- Skinless cod fillet 1 x 7-ounce
- Red onion, sliced 1/8 cup
- Celery, sliced 3/8 cup
- Garlic cloves, finely sliced 2
- Thai chili, finely sliced 1
- Finely sliced fresh ginger 1 teaspoon
- Green beans 3/8 cup
- Kale, roughly chopped 3/4 cup
- Sesame seeds 1 teaspoon
- Parsley, roughly chopped 2 tablespoons
- Tamari 1 tablespoon
- Buckwheat 1/4 cup
- Ground turmeric 1 teaspoon

Direction
1. Blend the oil with the mirin, miso and 1 teaspoon. Massage the cod all over and consider leaving for thirty min to marinate. Heat the oven up to 220 ° C (425oF).
2. Cook the cod for ten minutes.
3. In the meantime, heat the residual oil to a large skillet or wok. Stir-fry the onion for another few minutes, then bring the celery, chili, garlic, ginger, green beans, and kale. Toss and roast till the kale is roasted through and crispy. To help the frying process you might have to bring a little water to the skillet.

4. Fry the buckwheat along with the turmeric as per the manufacturer's guidelines.
5. To the stir-fry insert the parsley, sesame seeds, and tamari and represent with buckwheat and salmon.

Nutrition: 331 Calories 21g Fat 17g Protein

Superfood Salad

Preparation Time: 19 minutes
Cooking Time: 0 minutes
Serving: 2

Ingredients
- Arugula 1 3/4 ounces
- Endive leaves 1 3/4 ounces
- Smoked salmon slices 3 1/2 ounces
- Avocado, peeled, stoned, and sliced 1/2 cup
- Celery including leaves, sliced 1/2 cup
- Red onion, sliced 1/8 cup
- Walnuts, chopped 1/8 cups
- Capers 1 tablespoon
- Large Medjool date, pitted and chopped 1
- Extra-virgin olive oil 1 tablespoon
- Juice of lemon ¼
- Parsley, chopped 1/4 cup

Direction
1. Position the leaf of salad on a tray, or in a plastic bucket. Blend all the rest of the ingredients and represent over the foliage.

Nutrition: 307 Calories 17g Fat 6g Protein

Smoked Salmon Pasta

Preparation Time: 14 minutes
Cooking Time: 23 minutes
Serving: 4

Ingredients
- Extra virgin olive oil 2 tablespoons
- Red onion, finely sliced 1
- Garlic cloves, finely sliced 2
- Thai chilies, finely sliced 2
- Cherry tomatoes, cut in half 1 cup
- White wine 1/2 cup
- Buckwheat pasta 9 to 11 ounces
- Smoked salmon 9 ounces
- Capers 2 tablespoons
- Juice of lemon ½
- Arugula 2 ounces
- Parsley, chopped 1/4 cup

Direction
1. In a broiler pan start cooking one teaspoon of the oil over moderate flame. Stir in the onion, garlic, chili, and fry till smooth but not dark brown.
2. Start adding the tomatoes and permit to bake for one or two minutes. To minimize by half, append the white wine and bubble.
3. Bake the pasta in hot water with one tablespoon of oil for eight to ten minutes based on whether you like it to serve, then rinse.
4. Split the salmon into pieces and apply the capers, lemon juice, arugula, parsley, and the tomato into saucepan. Insert the sauce, blend together, and eat straight away. Sprinkle some oil over top.

Nutrition: 334 Calories 21g Fat 13g Protein

Vietnamese Turmeric Fish with Herbs & Mango Sauce

Preparation Time: 23 minutes
Cooking time: 34 minutes
Serving: 4

Ingredients
- Fresh cod fish 1 ¼ lbs.
- Coconut oil in pan and fry the fish 2 tablespoons
- Sea salt to taste

Fish marinade
- Turmeric powder 1 tablespoon
- Sea salt 1 teaspoon
- Chinese cooking wine 1 tablespoon
- Minced ginger 2 teaspoons
- Olive oil 2 tablespoons

Infused Scallion and Dill Oil
- Scallions 2 cups
- Fresh dill 2 cups
- Sea salt to taste

Mango dipping sauce
- Medium sized ripe mango 1
- Rice vinegar 2 tablespoons
- Juice of lime ½
- Garlic clove 1
- Dry red chili pepper 1 teaspoon

Direction
1. Marinate the fish for one hour or as long as it is overnight.

2. Add all ingredients in a mixing bowl under "Mango Dipping Sauce," and combine until quality is obtained.

For the Fish:

3. Cook 2 tablespoons of coconut oil at high temperature in a big, nonstick skillet. Add the pre-marinated fish if hot
4. A loud sizzle should be heard, upon which you can reduce the heat to moderate heat.
5. Do not turn or relocate the fish till after, about 5 minutes. Top with a tablespoon of sea salt.
6. When the fish is in golden brown, move the fish gently on the other side on cook. Transmit onto a large plate once it's accomplished.

For Scallion and Dill Infused Oil:

7. Just use rest of the oil over medium to high heat in the frying pan, stir in 2 cups of scallions and 2 cups of dill. Remove from the heat once the scallions and dill are introduced. Start giving them a delicate flip, about fifteen seconds, till the scallions and dill simmered. Season with a sprinkle of salt at sea.
8. Plop the scallion, dill and infused oil over the fish and represent fresh cilantro, lime, and nuts with mango sauce.

Nutrition: 471 Calories 31g Fat 21g Protein

Salmon Sirt Super Salad

Preparation Time: 13 minutes
Cooking Time: 0 minute
Serving: 2

Ingredients

- Rocket 50g
- Chicory leaves 50g
- Smoked salmon slices 100g
- Avocado 80g
- Celery 40g
- Red onion 20g
- Walnuts, finely sliced 15g
- Capers 1 tbs
- Large Medjool date 1
- Extra-virgin olive oil 1 tbs
- Juice of lemon ¼
- Parsley, finely sliced 10g
- Celery leaves or lovage, finely sliced 10g

Direction

1. Organize the leaves of the salad over a serving dish. Blend all the rest of the ingredients and represent over the leaves.

Nutrition: 349 Calories 26g Fat 13g Protein

Smoke Salmon with Egg

Preparation Time: 17 minutes
Cooking Time: 8 minutes
Serving: 1

Ingredients

- 2 medium eggs
- 100 g / 3.5 oz of smoked salmon, sliced
- 1/2 teaspoon capers
- 10 g / 0.35 oz of chopped rocket
- 1 teaspoon minced parsley
- 1 teaspoon of extra virgin olive oil

Direction

1. Crack eggs and beat well. Add salmon, capers, arugula and parsley.
2. Cook olive oil in a non-stick pan until it is hot but not smoking. Fill egg mix and lay it out around the pan equally.
3. Reduce the heat and let the omelet cook. Fold the tortilla in half to serve.
4. Heat an ovenproof skillet until hot, then add the marinated chicken and cook for 2 minutes on both sides, until lightly browned, then transfer to the oven for 8-10 minutes. Take out from the oven, wrap with foil and let rest for 5 minutes before serving.
5. Meanwhile, cook the black cabbage in a steamer for 5 minutes. Fry the red onions and ginger in a little oil until soft but not colored, then add the cooked cabbage and fry for another minute.

Nutrition: 291Calories 19g Fat 6g Protein

Stir-Fried Greens, Sesame & Cod

Preparation time: 16 minutes
Cooking Time: 11 minutes
Serving: 2

Ingredients:

- 20 g / 0.70 oz miso
- 1 tbsp mirin
- 1 tbsp extra virgin olive oil
- 200 g / 7 oz skinless cod fillet
- 20 g / 0.70 oz red onion, sliced
- 40 g / 1.4 oz celery, sliced

- 1 garlic clove, finely chopped
- 1 bird's eye chili, finely chopped
- 1 tsp finely chopped fresh ginger
- 60 g / 2.1 oz green beans
- 50 g / 1.7 oz kale, roughly chopped
- 1 tsp sesame seeds
- 5g / 1 tsp parsley, roughly chopped
- 1 tbsp tamari
- 30 g / 1 oz buckwheat
- 1 tsp ground turmeric

Direction
1. Blend miso, mirin, and 1 teaspoon of the oil. Brush all over the cod and marinate for 30 minutes. Set oven to 220°C/gas 7.
2. Bake the cod for 10 minutes.
3. Prep a frying pan with the remaining oil. Cook onion then mix celery, garlic, chili, ginger, green beans, and kale.
4. Cook the buckwheat following the packet's instructions for 3 minutes and sprinkle turmeric
5. Stir the sesame seeds, parsley, and tamari to the stir-fry and serve with the greens and fish.

Nutrition: 321 Calories 19g Fat 9g Protein

Turmeric Baked Salmon

Preparation time: 23 minutes
Cooking time: 14 minutes
Serving: 2

Ingredients
- 125-150 g / 4.5- 5.5 oz Skinned Salmon
- 1 tsp Extra virgin olive oil
- 1 tsp ground turmeric
- ¼ Juice of a lemon
- For the spicy celery
- 1 tsp Extra virgin olive oil
- 40 g / 1.4 oz Red onion, finely chopped
- 60 g / 2 oz Tinned green lentils
- 1 Garlic clove, finely chopped
- 1 cm fresh ginger, finely chopped
- 1 Bird's eye chili, finely chopped
- 150 g / 1.7 oz Celery, cut into 2cm lengths
- 1 tsp Mild curry powder
- 130 g / 4.5 oz Tomato, cut into eight wedges
- 100 ml / ½ cup Chicken or vegetable stock
- 1 tbsp Chopped parsley

Direction
1. Heat oven to 200 ° C.
2. Start with hot celery. Pre-heat frying pan over medium-low heat, add the olive oil, then the onion, garlic, ginger, chili and celery. Fry for 2 minutes, then add the curry powder and cook for another minute.
3. Add the tomatoes, then the broth and lentils and simmer for 10 minutes.
4. Blend turmeric, oil, and lemon juice and rub the salmon. Situate on a baking sheet and cook for 9 minutes.
5. Combine parsley through the celery and serve with the salmon.

Nutrition: 328 Calories 21g Fat 13g Protein

VEGETABLE RECIPES

Potato Carrot Salad

Preparation Time: 17 minutes
Cooking Time: 11 minutes
Servings: 6

Ingredients:
- Water
- Six potatoes, sliced into cubes
- Three carrots, sliced into cubes
- One tablespoon milk
- One tablespoon Dijon mustard
- ¼ cup mayonnaise
- Pepper to taste
- Two teaspoons fresh thyme, chopped
- One stalk celery, chopped
- Two scallions, chopped
- One slice turkey bacon, cooked crispy and crumbled

Directions:
1. Fill your pot with water.
2. Place it over medium-high heat.
3. Boil the potatoes and carrots for 10 to 15 minutes or until tender.
4. Drain and let cool.
5. In a bowl, mix the milk mustard, mayo, pepper, and thyme.
6. Stir in the potatoes, carrots, and celery.
7. Coat evenly with the sauce.
8. Cover and refrigerate for 4 hours.
9. Top with the scallions and turkey bacon bits before serving.

Nutrition: 106 Calories 5.3g Fat 2g Protein

High Protein Salad

Preparation Time: 6 minutes
Cooking Time: 7 minutes
Servings: 4

Ingredients:
Salad:
- One 15-oz can green kidney beans
- 2 4 tbsp capers
- 3 4 handfuls arugula
- 4 15-oz can lentils

Dressing:
- 5 1 tbsp caper brine
- 6 1 tbsp tamari
- 7 1 tbsp balsamic vinegar
- 8 2 tbsp peanut butter
- 9 2 tbsp hot sauce
- 10 1 tbsp tahini

Directions:
For the dressing:
1. In a bowl, stir together all the materials until they come together to form a smooth dressing.

For the salad:
2. Mix the beans, arugula, capers, and lentils. Top with the dressing and serve.

Nutrition: 205 Calories 2g Fat 13g Protein

Vegan Wrap with Apples and Spicy Hummus

Preparation Time: 12 minutes
Cooking Time: 0 minutes
Servings: 2

Ingredients:
- One tortilla
- 6-7 tbsp Spicy Hummus (mix it with a few tbsp of salsa)
- Only some leaves of fresh spinach or romaine lettuce
- 1 tsp fresh lemon juice
- 1½ cups broccoli slaw
- ½ apple, sliced thin
- 4 tsp dairy-free plain unsweetened yogurt
- Salt and pepper

Directions:
1. Mix the yogurt and the lemon juice with the broccoli slaw. Add the salt and a dash of pepper for taste. Mix well and set aside.
2. Lay the tortilla flat.
3. Spread the spicy hummus over the tortilla.
4. Lay the lettuce down on the hummus.
5. On one half, pile the broccoli slaw on the lettuce.
6. Place the apple slices on the slaw.
7. Fold the sides of the tortilla up, starting with the end that has the apple and the slaw. Roll tightly.
8. Cut it in half and serve.

Nutrition: 205 Calories 2g Fat 12g Protein

Rice and Veggie Bowl

Preparation Time: 7 minutes

Cooking Time: 12 minutes
Servings: 6
Ingredients:
- 2 tbsp coconut oil
- 1 tsp ground cumin
- 1 tsp ground turmeric
- 1 tsp chili powder
- One red bell pepper, chopped
- 1 tsp tomato paste
- One bunch of broccolis, cut into bite-sized florets with short stems
- 1 tsp salt, to taste
- One large red onion, sliced
- Two garlic cloves, minced
- One head of cauliflower, sliced into bite-sized florets
- 2 cups cooked rice
- Newly ground black pepper to taste

Directions:
1. Heat the coconut grease over medium-high heat in a large pan
2. Wait until the oil is hot, stir in the turmeric, cumin, chili powder, salt, and tomato paste.
3. Cook the content for 1 minute. Stir repeatedly until the spices are fragrant.
4. Add the garlic and onion. Sauté for 3 minutes.
5. Add the broccoli, cauliflower, and bell pepper. Cover the pot. Cook for 3 to 4 minutes and stir occasionally.
6. Add the cooked rice. Stir so it will combine well with the vegetables—Cook for 2 to 3 minutes. Stir until the rice is warmed through.
7. Check the seasoning. And make adjustments to taste if desired.
8. Decrease heat and cook on low for 2 to 3 more minutes so the flavors will meld.
9. Serve with freshly ground black pepper.

Nutrition: 260 Calories 9g Fat 9g Protein

Cucumber Tomato Chopped Salad

Preparation Time: 18 minutes
Cooking Time: 0 minutes
Servings: 6
Ingredients:
- ½ cup light mayonnaise
- One tablespoon lemon juice
- One tablespoon fresh dill, chopped
- One tablespoon chive, chopped
- ½ cup feta cheese, crumbled
- Salt and pepper to taste
- One red onion, chopped
- One cucumber, diced
- One radish, diced
- Three tomatoes, diced
- Chives, chopped

Directions:
1. Combine the mayo, lemon juice, fresh dill, chives, feta cheese, salt, and pepper in a bowl.
2. Mix well.
3. Stir in the onion, cucumber, radish, and tomatoes.
4. Coat evenly.
5. Garnish with the chopped chives.

Nutrition: 187 Calories 16.7g Fat 3.3g Protein

Zucchini Pasta Salad

Preparation Time: 6 minutes
Cooking Time: 0 minutes
Servings: 15
Ingredients:
- Five tablespoons olive oil
- Two teaspoons Dijon mustard
- Three tablespoons red-wine vinegar
- One clove garlic, grated
- Two tablespoons fresh oregano, chopped
- One shallot, chopped
- ¼ teaspoon red pepper flakes
- 16 oz. zucchini noodles
- ¼ cup Kalamata olives pitted
- 3 cups cherry tomatoes, sliced in half
- ¾ cup Parmesan cheese shaved

Directions:
1. Mix the olive oil, Dijon mustard, red wine vinegar, garlic, and oregano, shallot, and red pepper flakes in a bowl.
2. Stir in the zucchini noodles.
3. Sprinkle on top the olives, tomatoes, and Parmesan cheese.

Nutrition: 299 Calories 27g Fat 7g Protein

Egg Avocado Salad

Preparation Time: 14 minutes
Cooking Time: 0 minutes
Servings: 4

Ingredients:
- One avocado
- Six hard-boiled eggs, peeled and chopped
- One tablespoon mayonnaise
- Two tablespoons freshly squeezed lemon juice
- ¼ cup celery, chopped
- Two tablespoons chives, chopped
- Salt and pepper to taste

Directions:
1. Add the avocado to a large bowl.
2. Mash the avocado using a fork.
3. Stir in the egg and mash the eggs.
4. Add the mayo, lemon juice, celery, chives, salt, and pepper.
5. Chill in the refrigerator. Wait for at least 30 minutes before serving.

Nutrition: 224 Calories 19g Fat 10.6g Protein

Arugula Salad
Preparation Time: 17 minutes
Cooking Time: 0 minutes
Servings: 4

Ingredients:
- 6 cups fresh arugula leaves
- 2 cups radicchio, chopped
- ¼ cup low-fat balsamic vinaigrette
- ¼ cup pine nuts, toasted and chopped

Directions:
1. Arrange the arugula leaves in a serving bowl.
2. Sprinkle the radicchio on top.
3. Drizzle with the vinaigrette.
4. Sprinkle the pine nuts on top.

Nutrition: 85 Calories 6.6g Fat 2.2g Protein

Sautéed Cabbage
Preparation Time: 9 minutes
Cooking Time: 14 minutes
Servings: 8

Ingredients:
- ¼ cup butter
- One onion, sliced thinly
- One head cabbage, sliced into wedges
- Salt and pepper to taste
- Crumbled crispy bacon bits

Directions:
1. Cook butter to a pan over medium-high heat.
2. Cook the onion for 1 minute, stirring frequently.
3. Season with the salt and pepper.
4. Add the cabbage then stir it for 12 minutes.
5. Sprinkle with the crispy bacon bits.

Nutrition: 77 Calories 5.9g Fat 1.3g Protein

Cucumber Edamame Salad
Preparation Time: 6 minutes
Cooking Time: 9 minutes
Servings: 2

Ingredients:
- 3 tbsp. Avocado oil
- 1 cup cucumber, sliced into thin rounds
- ½ cup fresh sugar snap peas cut up or whole
- ½ cup fresh edamame
- ¼ cup radish, sliced
- One large avocado, peeled, pitted, sliced
- One nori sheet, crumbled
- 2 tsp. Roasted sesame seeds
- 1 tsp. Salt

Directions:
1. Make a medium-sized pot filled halfway with water to a boil over medium-high heat.
2. Add the sugar snaps and cook them for about 2 minutes.
3. Remove the pot off the heat, drain the excess water, transfer the sugar snaps to a medium-sized bowl, and set aside.
4. Fill the pot with water again, add the teaspoon of salt and bring to a boil over medium-high heat.
5. Add the edamame to the pot and let them cook for about 6 minutes.
6. Take the pot off the heat, drain the excess water, transfer the soybeans to the bowl with sugar snaps, and cool down for about 5 minutes.
7. Combine all ingredients, except for the nori crumbs and roasted sesame seeds, in a medium-sized bowl.
8. Delicately stir, using a spoon, until all ingredients are evenly coated in oil.
9. Top the salad along with the nori crumbs and roasted sesame seeds.
10. Shift the bowl to the fridge and allow the salad to cool for at least 30 minutes.

11. Serve chilled and enjoy!

Nutrition: 409 Calories 39g Fats 7.6g Protein

Garden Patch Sandwiches on Multigrain Bread

Preparation Time: 17 minutes
Cooking Time: 0 minutes
Servings: 4

Ingredients:
- 1pound extra-firm tofu drained and patted dry
- One medium red bell pepper, finely chopped
- One celery rib, finely chopped
- Three green onions, minced
- A quarter cup shelled sunflower seeds
- A half cup vegan mayonnaise, homemade or store-bought
- A half teaspoon salt
- A half teaspoon celery salt
- A quarter teaspoon freshly ground black pepper
- Eight slices whole grain bread
- 4 (1/4-inch) slices ripe tomato
- Four lettuce leaves

Directions:
1. Grind the tofu put it in a large bowl. Add the bell pepper, celery, green onions, and sunflower seeds. Stir in the mayonnaise, salt, celery salt, and pepper and mix until well combined.
2. Toast the bread, if desired. Spread the mixture evenly onto four slices of the bread. Top each with a tomato slice, lettuce leaf, and the remaining bread. Chop the sandwiches diagonally in half and serve.

Nutrition: 9g Protein 25g Fats 399 Calories

Garden Salad Wraps

Preparation Time: 18 minutes
Cooking Time: 12 minutes
Servings: 4

Ingredients:
- Six tablespoons olive oil
- 1-pound extra-firm tofu, drained, patted dry, and cut into 1/2-inch strips
- One tablespoon soy sauce
- A quarter cup apple cider vinegar
- One teaspoon yellow or spicy brown mustard
- A half teaspoon salt
- A quarter teaspoon freshly ground black pepper
- 3 cups shredded romaine lettuce
- Three ripe Roma tomatoes, finely chopped
- One large carrot, shredded
- One medium English cucumber, peeled and chopped
- 1/3 cup minced red onion
- A quarter cup sliced pitted green olives
- 4 (10-inch) whole-grain flour tortillas or lavash flatbread

Directions:
1. In a large frypan, heat two tablespoons of the oil over medium heat. Add the tofu. Cook it until golden brown, about 10 minutes. Sprinkle with soy sauce and set aside to cool. Combine the vinegar, mustard, salt, and pepper with the remaining four tablespoons oil, stirring to blend well. Set aside. Mix the lettuce, tomatoes, carrot, cucumber, onion, and olives. Pour on the dressing and flip to coat.
2. To assemble wraps, place one tortilla on a work surface and spread with about one-quarter of the salad. Place a few strips of tofu on the tortilla and roll up tightly. Slice in half

Nutrition: 89 Calories 8g Fat 4g Protein

Marinated Mushroom Wraps

Preparation Time: 14 minutes
Cooking Time: 0 minutes
Servings: 2

Ingredients:
- Three tablespoons soy sauce
- Three tablespoons fresh lemon juice
- 1A half tablespoons toasted sesame oil
- Two portobello mushroom caps
- One ripe Hass avocado pitted and peeled
- 2 cups fresh baby spinach leaves
- One medium red bell pepper
- One ripe tomato, chopped
- Salt and freshly ground black pepper

Directions;
1. Combine the soy sauce, two tablespoons of the lemon juice, and the oil. Add the portobello strips, toss to combine, and marinate for 1 hour or overnight. Drain the mushrooms and set aside.
2. Mash the avocado with the remaining one tablespoon of lemon juice.
3. To assemble wraps, place one tortilla on a work surface and spread with some of the mashed avocados. Topmost with a layer of baby spinach leaves.
4. In the lower third of each tortilla, arrange strips of the soaked mushrooms and some bell pepper strips. Sprinkle with the tomato and salt and black pepper to taste. Roll up tightly and cut in half diagonally. Repeat with the remaining ingredients and serve.

Nutrition: 89 Calories 8g Fat 4g Protein

Tamari Toasted Almonds

Preparation Time: 3 minutes
Cooking Time: 9 minutes
Servings: 2
Ingredients:
- ½ cup raw almonds, or sunflower seeds
- Two tablespoons tamari or soy sauce
- One teaspoon toasted sesame oil

Directions:
1. Preparing the ingredients.
2. Preheat dry skillet at medium-high heat, and then add the almonds, stirring very frequently to keep them from burning. Once the almonds are toasted, 7 to 8 minutes for almonds, or 3 to 4 minutes for sunflower seeds, pour the tamari and sesame oil into the hot skillet and stir to coat.
3. You can turn off the heat, and as the almonds cool, the tamari mixture will stick to and dry on the nuts.

Nutrition: 89 Calories 8g Fat 4g Protein

Peppers and Hummus

Preparation Time: 18 minutes
Cooking Time: 0 minutes
Servings: 4
Ingredients:
- One 15-ounce can chickpeas, drained and rinsed
- Juice of 1 lemon or one tablespoon prepared lemon juice
- ¼ cup tahini
- Three tablespoons olive oil
- ½ teaspoon ground cumin
- One tablespoon water
- ¼ teaspoon paprika
- One red bell pepper, sliced
- One green bell pepper, sliced
- One orange bell pepper, sliced

Directions:
1. In a food processor, mix chickpeas, lemon juice, tahini, two tablespoons of olive oil, cumin, and water.
2. A process on high speed until blended, about 30 seconds: scoop the hummus into a bowl and pour the remaining tablespoon of olive oil. Sprinkle with paprika. If desires, serve with sliced bell peppers.

Nutrition: 89 Calories 8g Fat 4g Protein

Baby Spinach Snack

Preparation Time: 12 minutes
Cooking Time: 13 minutes
Servings: 3
Ingredients:
- 2 cups baby spinach, washed
- A pinch of black pepper
- ½ tablespoon olive oil
- ½ teaspoon garlic powder

Directions:
1. Spread the baby spinach on a lined baking sheet, add oil, black pepper and garlic powder, toss a bit, introduce in the oven, bake at 350 degrees F for 10 minutes, divide into bowls and serve as a snack.

Nutrition: 125 calories 4g fat 2g protein

Bacon Potato Bites

Preparation Time: 17 minutes
Cooking Time: 22 minutes
Servings: 5
Ingredients:
- 1 potato
- 2 bacon slices
- 1 small avocado

Directions:
1. Spread potato slices on a lined baking sheet, spray with cooking oil, situate in the oven at 350 degrees F, bake for 20

minutes, arrange on a platter, top each slice with avocado and crumbled bacon and serve as a snack.

Nutrition: 187 calories 14g fat 16g protein

Dill Bell Pepper Snack Bowls

Preparation Time: 14 minutes
Cooking Time: 0 minutes
Servings: 4

Ingredients:
- 2 tablespoons dill, chopped
- 1 yellow onion, chopped
- 1 pound multi colored bell peppers
- 3 tablespoons olive oil
- 2 and ½ tablespoons white vinegar
- Black pepper to the taste

Directions:
1. In a salad bowl, mix bell peppers with onion, dill, pepper, oil and vinegar, toss to coat, divide into small bowls and serve as a snack.

Nutrition: 120 calories 3g fat 3g protein

Spicy Pumpkin Seeds Bowls

Preparation Time: 13 minutes
Cooking Time: 8 minutes
Servings: 6

Ingredients:
- ½ tablespoon chili powder
- ½ teaspoon cayenne pepper
- 2 cups pumpkin seeds
- 2 teaspoons lime juice

Directions:
1. Spread pumpkin seeds on a lined baking sheet, add lime juice, cayenne and chili powder, toss well, introduce in the oven, roast at 275 degrees F for 20 minutes, divide into small bowls and serve as a snack.

Nutrition: 170 calories 2g fat 6g protein

Apple and Pecans Bowls

Preparation Time: 14 minutes
Cooking Time: 0 minutes
Servings: 4

Ingredients:
- 4 big apples, cored, peeled and cubed
- 2 teaspoons lemon juice
- ¼ cup pecans, chopped

Directions:
1. Incorporate apples with lemon juice and pecans, toss, divide into small bowls and serve as a snack.

Nutrition: 120 calories 4g fat 3g protein

Zucchini Bowls

Preparation Time: 12 minutes
Cooking Time: 23 minutes
Servings: 12

Ingredients:
- Cooking spray
- ½ cup dill, chopped
- 1 egg
- ½ cup whole wheat flour
- Black pepper to the taste
- 1 yellow onion, chopped
- 2 garlic cloves, minced
- 3 zucchinis, grated

Directions:
1. In a bowl, mix zucchinis with garlic, onion, flour, pepper, egg and dill, stir well, shape small bowls out of this mix, arrange them on a lined baking sheet, grease them with some cooking spray, bake at 400 degrees F for 20 minutes, flipping them halfway, divide them into bowls and serve as a snack.

Nutrition: 120 calories 1g fat 6g protein

Cheesy Mushrooms Caps

Preparation Time: 14 minutes
Cooking time: 31 minutes
Servings: 20

Ingredients:
- 20 white mushroom caps
- 1 garlic clove, minced
- 3 tablespoons parsley, chopped
- 2 yellow onions, chopped
- Black pepper to the taste
- ½ cup low-fat parmesan, grated
- ¼ cup low-fat mozzarella, grated
- A drizzle of olive oil
- 2 tablespoons non-fat yogurt

Directions:
1. Pre-heat pan with some oil over medium heat, add garlic and onion, stir, cook for 10 minutes and transfer to a bowl.

2. Add black pepper, garlic, parsley, mozzarella, parmesan and yogurt, stir well, stuff the mushroom caps with this mix, arrange them on a lined baking sheet, bake in the oven at 400 degrees F for 20 minutes and serve them as an appetizer.

Nutrition: 120 calories 1g fat 7g protein

Mozzarella Cauliflower Bars

Preparation Time: 12 minutes
Cooking Time: 41 minutes
Servings: 12
Ingredients:
- 1 big cauliflower head, riced
- ½ cup low-fat mozzarella cheese, shredded
- ¼ cup egg whites
- 1 teaspoon Italian seasoning
- Black pepper to the taste

Directions:
1. Spread the cauliflower rice on a lined baking sheet, cook in the oven at 375 degrees F for 20 minutes, transfer to a bowl, add black pepper, cheese, seasoning and egg whites, stir well, spread into a rectangle pan and press well on the bottom.
2. Introduce in the oven at 375 degrees F, bake for 20 minutes, cut into 12 bars and serve as a snack.

Nutrition: 140 calories 1g fat 6g protein

Garlic Lovers Hummus

Preparation Time: 2 minutes
Cooking Time: 0 minute
Servings: 12
Ingredients:
- 3 tbsps. Freshly squeezed lemon juice
- All-purpose salt-free seasoning
- 3 tbsps. Sesame tahini
- 4 garlic cloves
- 15 oz. no-salt-added garbanzo beans
- 2 tbsps. Olive oil

Directions:
1. Drain garbanzo beans and rinse well.
2. Situate all the ingredients in a food processor and pulse until smooth.
3. Serve immediately or cover and refrigerate until serving.

Nutrition: 103 Calories 5g Fat: 4g Protein

Spinach and Kale Mix

Preparation Time: 5 minutes
Cooking Time: 0 minute
Servings: 4
Ingredients:
- 2 chopped shallots
- 1 c. no-salt-added and chopped canned tomatoes
- 2 c. baby spinach
- 2 minced garlic cloves
- 5 c. torn kale
- 1 tbsp. olive oil

Direction:
1. Warmup a pan with the oil over medium-high heat, add the shallots, stir and sauté for 5 minutes.
2. Add the spinach, kale and the other ingredients, toss, cook for 10 minutes more, divide between plates and serve.

Nutrition: 89 Calories 3.7g Fat 3.6g Protein

Turmeric Carrots

Preparation Time: 11 minutes
Cooking Time: 41 minutes
Servings: 4
Ingredients:
- 1-pound baby carrots, peeled
- 1 tablespoon olive oil
- 2 spring onions, chopped
- 2 tablespoons balsamic vinegar
- 2 garlic cloves, minced
- 1 teaspoon turmeric powder
- 1 tablespoon chives, chopped
- ¼ teaspoon cayenne pepper
- A pinch of salt and black pepper

Directions:
1. Arrange carrots in a baking sheet with parchment paper, toss oil, spring onions and the other ingredients, then bake at 380 degrees F for 40 minutes. Serve

Nutrition: 79 calories 3.8g fat 1g protein

Spinach Mix

Preparation Time: 13 minutes
Cooking Time: 14 minutes
Servings: 4
Ingredients:
- 1-pound baby spinach
- 1 yellow onion, chopped

- 1 tablespoon olive oil
- 1 tablespoon lemon juice
- 2 garlic cloves, minced
- A pinch of cayenne pepper
- ¼ teaspoon smoked paprika
- A pinch of salt and black pepper

Directions:
1. Preheat pan with the oil over medium-high heat, cook onion and the garlic for 2 minutes.
2. Add the spinach and the other ingredients, toss, cook over medium heat for 10 minutes, divide between plates and serve as a side dish.

Nutrition: 71 calories 4g fat 3.7g protein

Orange Carrots

Preparation Time: 7 minutes
Cooking Time: 22 minutes
Servings: 4

Ingredients:
- 1-pound carrots, peeled and roughly sliced
- 1 yellow onion, chopped
- 1 tablespoon olive oil
- Zest of 1 orange, grated
- Juice of 1 orange
- 1 orange, peeled and cut into segments
- 1 tablespoon rosemary, chopped
- A pinch of salt and black pepper

Direction:
1. Warmup a pan with the oil over medium-high heat, add the onion and sauté for 5 minutes.
2. Add the carrots, the orange zest and the other ingredients, toss, cook over medium heat for 20 minutes more, divide between plates and serve.

Nutrition: 140 calories 3.9g fat 2.1g protein

Zucchini Pan

Preparation Time: 4 minutes
Cooking Time: 23 minutes
Servings: 4

Ingredients:
- 1-pound zucchinis, sliced
- 1 yellow onion, chopped
- 2 tablespoons olive oil
- 2 apples, peeled, cored and cubed
- 1 tomato, cubed
- 1 tablespoon rosemary, chopped
- 1 tablespoon chives, chopped

Direction:
1. With a pan, preheat oil on medium heat, cook onion for 3 minutes.
2. Cook zucchinis and the other ingredients at medium heat for 17 minutes then serve.

Nutrition: 170 calories 5g fat 7g protein

Stir-Fried Mushroom with Ginger

Preparation Time: 14 minutes
Cooking time: 27 minutes
Servings: 3

Ingredients:
- 1-lb. mushrooms
- 1-piece yellow onion
- 1 tbsp. ginger
- 1 tbsp. olive oil
- 2 tbsp. balsamic vinegar
- 2 garlic cloves
- 0.25 cup lime juice
- 2 tbsp. walnuts

Directions:
1. In a pan, cook oil over medium-high heat, sauté onion and ginger for 5 minutes.
2. Cook mushrooms and the other ingredients, at medium heat for 15 minutes more and serve.

Nutrition: 123 calories 3g fat 6g protein

Polenta Bake

Preparation Time: 7 minutes
Cooking Time: 27 minutes
Serving: 6

Ingredients
- One tablespoon of olive oil
- ½ diced medium-sized eggplant (if allergic, use mushrooms)
- ½ diced small sized zucchini
- ¼ teaspoon of salt
- ¼ cup of water
- ¼ teaspoon of freshly grounded pepper
- 5 ounces of baby spinach
- 1 cup of prepared marinara sauce
- ¼ cup of chopped fresh basil
- 7 ounces of prepared polenta
- 1 cup of shredded part-skim mozzarella
- Six tablespoons of cheese

Direction:
1. Preheat your oven to 232 C
2. Coat your baking dish with some cooking spray
3. Place a large nonstick skillet on medium-high heat.
4. Then add your diced eggplants, zucchini, salt, and pepper.
5. Allow the ingredients cook, but make sure you occasionally stir until the vegetables are soft and about to turn brown. This process should last 4-6 minutes. Don't let the vegetables burn.
6. Add your baby spinach. Let the spinach cook for about 3 minutes until it wilts. Stir only once.
7. Add your marinara sauce into the vegetables and stir. Let it heat for a minute or two,
8. Turn off the heat and stir in your basil.
9. Put polenta slices in your baking dish. Place them in a single layer. You can trim the slices to fit in the dish if necessary.
10. Sprinkle your cheese on the polenta
11. Top polenta with eggplant mixture. You can add more cheese.
12. Bake for 12-15 minutes until it's bubbling and the cheese has melted. Leave it for 5 minutes after baking before you serve.

Nutrition 2.7g Fats 4.1g Protein 201 Calories

Raw Carrot and Almond Loaf

Preparation Time: 18 minutes
Cooking Time: 7 minutes
Serving: 4

Ingredients
- 6-8 medium-sized fresh carrots
- Juice of ½ medium-sized lemon
- ½ cup of almonds
- Fresh and chopped Parsley
- Four tablespoons of tahini
- 40g plain flour (optional)
- 30g Coconut sugar or as much as you wish (optional)
- ¼ teaspoon of baking powder (optional)

Direction
1. Grate your carrots properly
2. Put the grated carrots in a food processor with an S blade.
3. Blend carrots and lemon in the food processor. Let them whizz properly.
4. Transfer the mixture into a bowl.
5. Whizz up almond into the processor. Almonds must be well-grounded.
6. Then, add the blended almonds and carrot mixture together.
7. Add your parsley and tahini and blend them all.
8. Transfer your mixture into a loaf thin. Bake for 7 minutes.
9. Cut into slices to serve. Serve as an appetizer.
10. If you wish to add flour, sugar, and baking powder, you should cover the mixture with foil and leave it to bake for up to 45 minutes.
11. Carrot and almond loaf can be served with cream cheese icing topping. But be careful; you don't want to take too much sugar.
12. For cream cheese toppings, mix one tablespoon of low-fat yogurt, 20g cream cheese, lemon juice, and sugar in a bowl. Put it in a refrigerator to freeze. Then serve when the baked loaf is ready.

Nutrition 7g Fats 6.5g Protein 103 Calories

Kale and Red Onion Dhal with Bucket Wheat

Preparation Time: 17 minutes
Cooking Time: 21 minutes
Serving: 5

Ingredients
- 160g of bucket wheat
- 100g of kale
- 200ml of water
- 160g of red lentils
- 400ml of coconut milk
- 2 cm of grated ginger cloves
- Two teaspoons of turmeric
- One seedless and finely chopped birds eye chili
- Three grated garlic cloves
- Two teaspoons of garam masala
- One sliced red onion

Direction
1. Place a deep saucepan on low heat. Add your olive oil and onions and allow it to

cook for 5 minutes. Your onions should soften and not turn brown.
2. Then, add your ginger, chili, and garlic.
3. Add turmeric, garam masala, and just a splash of water. Let it cook for another minute.
4. Next, you add lentils, coconut milk, and 200ml of water. To get the right measurement for your water, you can just pour water into the coconut milk can and then into the pan.
5. Mix your ingredients properly. Cook for 23 minutes more.
6. Then, add your kale, stir and cover it to cook for 5 minutes.
7. Cook your buckwheat in a medium-sized saucepan separately for 10 minutes before curry is ready. You can do this 15minutes before the curry is ready.
8. Serve bucket wheat and curry on a plate when they are ready.

Nutrition 12g Fats 3.4g Proteins 458 Calories

Kale with Lemon Tahini Dressing

Preparation Time: 18 minutes
Cooking Time: 0 minutes
Serving: 6
Ingredients
For your salad
- 250- 275g of curly kale
- one tablespoon of squeezed lemon juice
- ½ tablespoon of olive oil
- ½ tablespoon of toasted sesame oil
- one medium-sized carrot
- ½ tablespoon of pure maple syrup
- one medium-sized beet
- 2-3 tablespoons of pumpkin seeds.
- one tablespoon of hemp seeds (optional)
- A pinch of salt

For dressing
- three tablespoons of tahini
- one minced garlic clove
- three tablespoons of olive oil
- 80ml of squeezed lemon juice
- Salt and pepper

Direction
1. Remove the large stems from the curly kale. You can use Tuscan kale if you wish.
2. Squeeze your lemon juice separately. Make sure you pick out all the seeds. Since you will need lemon juice for dressing, you should get more than one lemon.
3. Make sure your carrot and beet are peeled and grated.
4. Begin preparation. Pour your kale into a large salad bowl. Add lemon juice, oil, maple syrup, salt, and garlic.
5. Massage the mixture gently with your hand. Continue massaging until kale is soft and wilting. This process should last for 3-5 minutes.
6. Give kale extra time to soften by setting the mixture aside to marinate for 15-20 minutes.
7. Prepare your dressing. In a smaller bowl, add tahini, lemon juice, garlic, olive oil, salt, and pepper. Whisk the mixture properly. Taste and adjust seasoning as you desire. Then set aside.
8. When the kale is ready, pour the dressing over the kale. Toss the salad until it is evenly coated.
9. Add grated carrot and beet and toss it again until it has mixed well. If you are using hemp seeds, make sure they are hulled and sprinkle them over the salad.

Nutrition 20g Fats 10g Protein 189 Calories

Broccoli and Kale Green Soup

Preparation Time: 18 minutes
Cooking Time: 31 minutes
Serving: 4
Ingredients
- 1 liter of stock
- one tablespoon of sunflower oil
- four sliced garlic cloves
- two thumb-sized ginger
- one teaspoon of ground coriander
- two pieces of fresh turmeric root
- ½ teaspoon of Himalayan salt
- 400g of roughly sliced courgette
- 170g of broccoli
- 200g of chopped kale
- A pack of parsley for garnish; don't cut all
- two limes, zest, and juice

Direction

1. Put your sunflower oil in a deep pan. Add garlic, coriander, ginger, turmeric, and salt. Then, fry for 2 minutes on medium heat. Stir so it doesn't burn.
2. Then add three tablespoons of water, so the spices don't get too dry,
3. Add courgette and mix well. Make sure you mix the courgette into the spices thoroughly. Allow it to coat well and cook for 3 minutes.
4. Add 400ml stock and allow it to simmer for 3 minutes. You can make stock by mixing two tablespoons of bouillon powder into boiling water.
5. Then, add your broccoli, lime juice, kale, and the remaining stock into the soup. Allow it to cook for 3-4 minutes.
6. Turn off the heat and add your roughly chopped parsley. Leave some whole leaves for garnish.
7. Fill your soup into a blender and blend on high speed.
8. Serve into four plates. Garnish with zest lime and whole parsley.

Nutrition 8g Fats 10g Protein 182 Calories

Butter Bean and Vegetable Korma

Preparation Time: 9 minutes
Cooking Time: 34 minutes
Serving: 4

Ingredients

- three normal-size cloves of garlic
- one onion
- one fresh chili
- ½ piece of fresh ginger, thumb size
- 750g sweet potatoes
- one medium tomato
- 250g frozen peas
- 100g green sugar snaps/beans
- 2 tbsp. oil
- 400g large leek
- 400ml water
- one tin (400ml) coconut milk
- 3 tbsp. soy sauce/tamari
- 1 tbsp. honey
- 2 tsp. ground cumin
- Juice of a lemon
- 2 tsp. ground coriander
- 1 tsp. ground turmeric
- 2 tsp. salt
- 4 tsp. medium curry powder
- ½ tsp. freshly ground black pepper
- Bunch of fresh coriander
- one tin (400g) butterbeans

Direction

1. Pour two tablespoons of oil into a huge saucepan. Chop the tomato, red onion and put them into the pan
2. Add the grated ginger, chili chopped garlic into the pan and have it cooked for about five minutes.
3. Prepare the leeks and sweet potato. Do not forget to include the leafy bits
4. Add the ground cumin, curry powder, turmeric, ground coriander, and black pepper to the pan.
5. Next, add 400 ml of water, one tin of coconut milk, two teaspoons of salt, the juice of 1 lemon, 1tablespoons of liquid sweetener, and three tablespoons of tamari (or soy sauce)
6. Add the leeks, sweet potato, and beans and have the mixture stewed until the sweet potatoes are cooked or for about 20 minutes.
7. Save a few peas for the purpose of garnishing and the rest of it inside. Also, add sugar snap peas. Serve!

Nutrition: 417 calories 19g fats 8g protein

Courgette Tortilla

Preparation Time: 8 minutes
Cooking Time: 21 minutes
Serving: 2

Ingredients

- 1 tbsp. olive oil
- one large coarsely grated courgette
- 1 tsp. harissa
- four large eggs
- 3 tbsps. reduced-fat hummus
- one large red pepper, torn into strips
- three pitted queen olives, quartered
- Handful coriander

Direction

1. Cook oil in a 20cm non-stick frying pan. Put the courgette and let it cook for some

minute while stirring it periodically until it softens.
2. Beat the eggs with the harissa and pour them into the pan.
3. Proceed to cook gently. Stir to let the egg that is uncooked flow onto the base of the pan.
4. When more than half has been cooked, do not touch it for about two minutes. Place a plate, then take back to the pan, facing the uncooked part down, to have the cooking completed.
5. Tip on top of a board and spread using the hummus to serve.
6. Scatter with the coriander, olives, and pepper.
7. Cut into quarters and eat cold or warm.

Nutrition: 317 calories 21g fat 13g protein

Almond Butter and Alfalfa Wraps

Preparation Time: 7 minutes
Cooking Time: 0 minutes
Servings: 1
Ingredients
- Juice of 1 lemon
- 4 tbsp. of almond nut butter
- three finely sliced radishes
- 2-3 carrots grated
- 1 cup of alfalfa sprouts
- Nori sheets or lettuce leaves
- Pepper and salt

Direction
1. Combine the almond butter with a sufficient amount of water and an ample amount of lemon juice so you will have a paste with your desired level of thickness.
2. Next, have the alfalfa sprouts and grated carrot mixed inside a bowl. Sprinkle with the remaining lemon juice that was set aside. Proceed to the season with pepper and salt to taste.
3. Using the almond butter, smear the nori sheets or lettuce leaves, depending on the one you are using. Top the resulting mixture with the alfalfa sprout mixture and carrot. Roll it up and serve. Enjoy!

Nutrition: 409 calories 17g fat 6g protein

Buckwheat Bean and Tomato Risotto

Preparation Time: 11 minutes
Cooking Time: 23 minutes
Servings: 4
Ingredients
- 2 tbsp. of butter or olive oil
- two cloves of chopped garlic
- eight ounces/225g buckwheat
- 400ml of vegetable stock or hot water
- eight ounces/225g broad beans
- ½ cup of sun-dried tomatoes inside an oil
- Juice of half a lemon
- 2 tbsp. of chopped coriander or basil
- two ounces/50g of toasted almonds
- Pepper and salt

Direction
1. Heat the butter or olive oil inside a frying pan. Include the garlic and allow it to cook for a period of one minute.
2. Next, place the buckwheat into the pan and have it stirred thoroughly. This is to allow the buckwheat to be coated in the oil.
3. After that, add the stock or hot water. Then close the frying pan and let it simmer for 10 minutes.
4. When you are done simmering, stir the broad beans in. Then proceed to cook until the beans are just tender, which should be for a few minutes.
5. After that, add the fresh herbs, lemon juice, sun-dried tomatoes, and almonds. Season with pepper and salt to taste. Serve and enjoy your meal!

Nutrition: 358 calories 21g fat 14g protein

Vegetable Curry with Tofu

Preparation Time: 14 minutes
Cooking Time: 20 minutes
Serving: 3
Ingredients
- ½ tbsp. rapeseed oil
- One large onion, chopped
- three cloves garlic, peeled and grated
- One large thumb (7cm) fresh ginger, peeled and grated
- One red chili, deseeded and thinly sliced
- ¼ tsp ground turmeric

- ¼ tsp cayenne pepper
- ½ tsp paprika
- ¼ tsp ground cumin
- ½ tsp salt
- 150g dried red lentils
- ½-liter boiling water
- 30g frozen soya edamame beans
- 100g firm tofu, chopped into cubes
- a tomato, roughly chopped
- Juice of 1 lime
- 100g kale leaves stalk removed and torn

Direction
1. Put the oil over low-medium heat in a heavy-bottom pan. Add the turmeric, cayenne, cumin, paprika, and oil. Remove and mix again before adding the red lentils.
2. Pour in the boiling water and cook for 10 minutes until the curry has a thick 'porridge' consistency, then reduce the heat and cook for another 20-30 minutes.
3. Add soya beans, tofu, and tomatoes and continue to cook for another 5 minutes. Add the juice of lime and kale leaves and cook until the kale is tender.

Nutrition 342 Calories 5g Fat 28g Protein

Sirt Food Mushroom Scramble Eggs

Preparation Time: 6 minutes
Cooking Time: 9 minutes
Serving: 4

Ingredients
- two eggs
- 1 tsp ground turmeric
- 1 tsp mellow curry powder
- 20g kale, generally slashed
- 1 tsp additional virgin olive oil
- ½ superior bean stews, daintily cut
- Bunch of catch mushrooms, meagerly cut
- 5g parsley, finely slashed

Direction
1. Blend the turmeric and curry powder and include a little water until you have accomplished light glue.
2. Steam the kale for 2–3 minutes.
3. Preheat oil in a skillet at medium heat and fry the bean stew and mushrooms for 2 minutes.
4. Include the eggs and flavor glue and cook over medium warmth at that point, add the kale and keep on cooking over medium heat for a further moment. At long last, include the parsley, blend well and serve.

Nutrition 158 Calories 9.96g Protein 10.9g Fat

Green Salad Skewers

Preparation Time: 17 minutes
Cooking Time: 0 minutes
Serving: 6

Ingredients
- Eight large black olives
- Eight cherry tomatoes
- One yellow pepper
- ½ red onion, chopped
- 100g cucumber, sliced
- 100g feta, chopped into 8
- Ingredients for the dressing
- two wooden skewers
- eight cherry tomatoes
- one tablespoon of extra virgin olive oil
- ½ lemons
- one teaspoon of balsamic vinegar
- ½ clove garlic, peeled and crushed
- Few basil leaves, finely chopped
- Few leaves oregano, finely chopped
- Salt
- Freshly ground black pepper

Direction
1. Let the wooden skewers get soaked for 30 minutes with water
2. The skewers then need to be filled with the salad ingredients.
3. Mix all the dressing ingredients in a bowl, then pour over the skewers.

Nutrition 236 Calories 46g Fat 7g Protein

Baked Potatoes with Spicy Chickpea Stew

Preparation Time: 9 minutes
Cooking Time: 38 minutes
Serving: 4

Ingredients
- One red onion, nicely chopped
- Two cloves- grated
- Grated ginger (1cm)
- One tablespoon, chili-flakes
- Turmeric one -tablespoon

- A sprinkle of water
- Nicely chopped tomatoes (2×200g)
- Cocoa powder (unsweetened) 1tbs
- Two tin of chickpeas (200g each ×2)
- Nicely chopped pepper in smaller sizes
- Parsley with garnish (one tablespoon)
- Salt
- Pepper

Direction
1. Get all ingredients ready.
2. Preheat oven, over an average heat/preferably 200 degree).
3. When heated to a desired extent, place baking potatoes and cooked to your desired satisfaction, preferably for one hour: to fifteen minutes.
4. Get a saucepan and placed in your olive oil alongside the chopped onion, and cooked till onions are soft.
5. Cook more for five minutes over average heat, adding your garlic, chili, and ginger with it.
6. Add water (a little splash), turmeric, and cook for some minutes (preferably 4-5 minutes).
7. At this stage, the tomatoes, pepper, (yellow), and cocoa powder will be added and cooked for 35 minutes over an average heat till its sauce and thick to an extent.
8. Add salt (a pinch of it), parsley (two tablespoons), and pepper (optional) when the stew is almost ready.
9. Stir and serve on potatoes (Baked).

Nutrition: 391 calories 27g fat 14g protein

Buckwheat Garden Salad

Preparation Time: 19 minutes
Cooking Time: 0 minutes
Serving: 3

Ingredients
- One cup of buckwheat
- Water, two cups
- Salt, half teaspoon
- Half cherry Lotte nicely diced
- Green olives, 12 preferably large
- Two nicely diced (yellow pepper)
- Smoothly chopped broccoli florets, one cup
- 50gram of walnuts, chopped
- Half cup of fresh dill, smoothly chopped
- One lime of juice
- Olive oil, one tablespoon
- Half teaspoon of black pepper

Direction
1. Get a saucepan, medium-size, and fill with small water to boil.
2. Salt, buckwheat groats will be added to the boiling water to cook till it absorbed the ingredients.
3. Allow the cooked buckwheat to cool for an hour before adding green olive, cherry Lotte, yellow bell pepper (diced), red onions, florets, chopped broccoli, and walnuts in a fitted bowl for thorough mixing.
4. Serve meal immediately after mixing or reserved for hours in a refrigerator.

Nutrition: 417 calories 29g fat 15g protein

Cucumber, Pineapple, Parsley, And Lemon Smoothie

Preparation Time: 7 minutes
Cooking Time: 0 minutes
Serving: 2

Ingredients
- A bunch of leaf parsley nicely chopped.
- Coconut water 3/4 cup.
- Half cucumber, nicely chopped.
- Two cups of frozen pineapple.
- A drip of liquid stevia (5 drops preferably)
- Ginger.

Direction
1. Ensure the ingredients are ready.
2. Get a blender, preferably a bigger blender.
3. Place ingredients in one at a time to blend all.
4. Blend ingredients over extremely high heat for three minutes till it's super creamy and smooth to serve.

Nutrition: 98 calories 11g fat 3g protein

Buckwheat Meatballs

Preparation Time: 14 minutes
Cooking Time: 18 minutes
Serving: 4

Ingredients:
- 100 grams of buckwheat;
- 1 whole egg;

- a clove of garlic;
- a bunch of parsley;
- nutmeg;
- breadcrumbs;
- salt and pepper.

Directions
1. Wash the buckwheat and transfer it to a pot. Let it toast for a few seconds, after which add about 250/300 ml of cold water, sprinkle salt, and cook for 23 minutes.
2. Chop a clove of garlic and put it in a pan with a drizzle of oil, add the buckwheat well drained from the remaining cooking water and let it flavor together for a few minutes. Transfer everything into a bowl and let it cool.
3. When the wheat is warm, add the slightly beaten egg, nutmeg, finely chopped parsley, a pinch of pepper, and mix well.
4. Now form some balls with the help of a spoon and roll them in breadcrumbs. Compact the meatballs by squeezing them between the palms of your hands and, at the same time, flatten them slightly at the poles.
5. Grease a pan with oil and cook the meatballs on both sides until they are golden brown. Serve them hot buckwheat meatballs accompanied by vegetables to taste.

Nutrition: 471 calories 16g fats 7g protein

Cabbage and Buckwheat Fritters

Preparation Time: 11 minutes
Cooking Time: 4 minutes
Serving: 3
Ingredients:
- 20 g grated cheese
- 50 g cabbage tops
- 1 egg
- 1 tablespoon Flour 00
- 1/2 shallot
- Extra virgin olive oil
- Salt

Directions
1. Clean the cabbage and choose the florets. Finely cut the shallot and situate in the pressure cooker with 1 tablespoon of oil and the cabbage florets.
2. Brown gently, add the buckwheat and twice as much saltwater or vegetable broth. Close the pan and cook for 15 minutes from the start of the hiss.
3. Open the pot and let the mixture cool down. Add the egg and add enough flour to obtain a homogeneous mixture with a moderately firm consistency.
4. If necessary, add salt to taste. With floured hands, form round meatballs and then crush them slightly to flatten them.
5. Place them in a baking tray and brush them with a drizzle of oil. Bake them in the oven for 15 minutes at about 200 °C (392 °F)

Nutrition: 391 calories 12g fat 6g protein

Buckwheat Salad with Artichokes

Preparation Time: 18 minutes
Cooking Time: 6 minutes
Serving: 4
Ingredients:
- 300 g buckwheat
- 200 g cherry tomatoes
- 5 artichokes
- 1 clove of garlic
- 1/2 cup large green olives
- fresh marjoram
- 5 tablespoons extra virgin olive oil
- salt
- 1 lemon

Directions
1. Using non-stick pan, toast the buckwheat grains, always stirring for 3 minutes, then boil salted water for 11 minutes. Drain and set aside.
2. Clean the artichokes: remove the outer leaves, trim them and remove the beard, cut them into segments, and throw them away as they are cleaned in water acidulated with lemon juice, so that they do not blacken.
3. In the meantime, brown the clove of garlic dressed lightly crushed in two tablespoons of oil.
4. When the artichokes are all hulled and cut, drain them and put them in the pan.

Brown them without burning, then lower the heat and cook until they have softened a bit; they must remain al dente. Remove the garlic clove and sprinkle with a little fresh marjoram.
5. Put the buckwheat in the pan with the artichokes, stir well, and cook for a couple of minutes to make it taste good. Turn off and set aside.
6. Rinse and chop the cherry tomatoes in 2, leaving them a little in a colander to drain the vegetation water.
7. Slice olives in half and remove the stone.
8. Incorporate the cherry tomatoes and olives with buckwheat, add more marjoram leaves, stir and let them flavor well covered, over low heat.

Nutrition: 341 calories 21g fat 15g protein

Pasta with Rocket Salad and Linseed

Preparation Time: 21 minutes
Cooking Time: 21 minutes
Serving: 4
Ingredients:
- 400 gr of whole meal pasta
- 1 bunch of washed and dried Rocket
- 1 tablespoon of peeled almonds
- 1 tablespoon Linseed
- 1/2 clove of Garlic
- 4 spoons of extra virgin olive oil
- 3 tablespoons of water (if necessary)
- A few drops of lemon juice
- Salt
- Pepper

Directions
1. First, wash the arugula and put it to dry on a kitchen cloth, then boil water and throw the dough;
2. In a mixer, add 1 tablespoon of linseed, 1 tablespoon of almonds, half a clove of garlic (without the sprout) and 4 tablespoons of oil;
3. Cut everything for a few minutes, if necessary, add a little water to make the pesto more fluid;
4. At this point add the rocket, a few drops of lemon juice, a pinch of salt and turn the mixer again for a few seconds, then add salt and pepper, and your pesto is ready;
5. Before draining the pasta, set aside some cooking water so that it can be used later, in case the pesto is too thick;
6. Once drained, put the pasta on the pot, season it with the pesto, and, if necessary, add a little cooking water previously-stored; continuing to stir for about a minute, and now your dish is ready to taste!

Nutrition: 401 calories 29g fat 17g protein

Sirt Yogurt

Preparation Time: 7 minutes
Cooking Time: 0 minutes
Serving: 1
Ingredients
- 125g mixed berries
- 150g Greek yogurt
- 25g of chopped walnuts
- 10g of dark chocolate (85 percent cocoa) grated

Directions
1. Put your favorite berries in a bowl and pour yogurt on top. Sprinkle them with nuts and chocolate.
2. For a vegan alternative, you can replace Greek yogurt with soy or coconut milk.

Nutrition: 297 calories 27g fat 11g protein

Sirt Pita Bread

Preparation Time: 14 minutes
Cooking Time: 17 minutes
Serving: 4
Ingredients
- 1 c. warm water
- 2 tsp. active dry yeast
- 1 tsp. granulated sugar
- 3 c. all-purpose flour, divided
- 1 tbsp. extra-virgin olive oil
- 1 1/2 tsp. kosher salt

Direction
1. Situate pizza stone or large cast iron skillet in your oven and preheat to 500 F. Mix warm water, yeast, and sugar until dissolved. Stir in ½ cup flour and set aside for 15 minutes
2. Combine oil, salt, and 2 cups flour (reserving ½ cup) until a shaggy mass

form. Sprinkle clean surface with some of reserved flour and knead for 7 minutes.
3. Situate dough in a clean large bowl and wrap with plastic. Keep aside in warm place for 1 hour.
4. Slightly dust a clean surface with flour. Press down dough and turn it out onto surface. Portion dough into 8 pieces and roll into balls. Seal with a towel for 10 minutes.
5. Working one simultaneously, roll each round into a ¼"-thick circle about 8" wide, dust dough with extra flour if it starts to stick.
6. Situate as many pitas that will fit on your skillet then bake 5 minutes. Repeat
7. Wrap baked pitas with a clean kitchen towel to keep warm.

Nutrition: 487 calories 26g fat 13g protein

Red Bean Sauce with Baked Potato

Preparation Time: 21 minutes
Cooking Time: 15 minutes
Serving: 1

Ingredients:
- 40g red onion, finely chopped
- 1 teaspoon of fresh ginger, finely chopped
- 1 clove of garlic, finely chopped
- 1 Bird's Eye chili pepper, finely chopped
- 1 teaspoon of extra virgin olive oil
- 1 teaspoon of turmeric powder
- 1 teaspoon of cumin powder
- 1 pinch of powdered cloves
- 1 pinch of cinnamon powder
- 1 medium potato 190g peeled
- 1 teaspoon of brown sugar
- 50g red pepper, stripped of stalks and seeds and coarsely chopped
- 150ml vegetable stock
- 1 tablespoon of cocoa powder
- 1 teaspoon of sesame seeds
- 2 teaspoons of peanut butter
- 150g canned red beans
- 5g chopped parsley

Directions
1. Set oven to 200 °C (392 °F).
2. Fry the onion, ginger, garlic, and chili pepper in oil in a medium pan over medium heat for about 12 minutes. Cook spices for 2 minutes.
3. Place the potato on a baking tray, put it in the hot oven and cook for 45-60 minutes
4. Add the peeled tomatoes, sugar, peppers, stock, cocoa powder, sesame seeds, peanut butter, and beans; and simmer for 45-60 minutes.
5. Finally, sprinkle with parsley.

Nutrition: 491 calories 31g fat 16g protein

Curly Kale with Sweet Potatoes

Preparation Time: 23 minutes
Cooking Time: 19 minutes
Serving: 1

Ingredients:
- 50g Curly Kale
- 200 g Sweet potatoes
- Red onion
- 1 teaspoon bird's eye chili pepper
- 2 tablespoons extra virgin olive oil
- Salt

Directions
1. Slice sweet potatoes into small cubes and put them in a pan with a drizzle of oil and the onion into small pieces.
2. Add salt. Once cooked, add the cut kale and chili pepper. Turn well until the kale is well withered. Continue cooking for another 5 minutes, always stirring with a ladle!

Nutrition: 391 calories 24g fat 9g protein

Buckwheat Pasta with Zucchini and Cherry Tomatoes

Preparation Time: 9 minutes
Cooking Time: 29 minutes
Serving: 2

Ingredients:
- 160 g buckwheat pasta
- 2 zucchinis
- 6 cherry tomatoes
- 1/2 red onion
- extra virgin olive oil
- halls

- bird's-eye chili

Directions
1. Fry the oil in a pan with the sliced onion and chili pepper.
2. When the onion has taken a little color, add the cherry tomatoes and zucchini slices; turn well and let cook with a lid on medium heat for about 10 minutes, turning occasionally.
3. Boil the salted water for the pasta, then drain the pasta.
4. Throw it directly into the sauce and fry everything in a pan for about a minute.

Nutrition: 458 calories 23g fats 18g protein

Pasta with Red Chicory and Walnuts

Preparation Time: 9 minutes
Cooking Time: 32 minutes
Serving: 1

Ingredients:
- 70 g buckwheat pasta
- 100 g red chicory
- 10 g extra virgin olive oil
- 20 g walnuts
- 30 g bacon cut into strips
- 10g Bird's eye chili minced
- Salt

Directions
1. Stew the red chicory in a saucepan with oil, and when it is cooked, add the walnut grains that you have previously browned with bacon cut into strips.
2. Cook pasta in salted water, strain it and add it to the mixture of red chicory and walnuts and sauté for a few seconds; finally, a sprinkling of chili.

Nutrition: 319 calories 15g fat 9g protein

Cabbage and Red Chicory Flan

Preparation Time: 13 minutes
Cooking Time: 18 minutes
Serving: 4

Ingredients:
- 800g cabbage
- 250g red chicory
- 100g red onions 100 g
- 3 tablespoons Extra virgin olive oil
- Salt
- Pepper
- 2 tablespoon breadcrumbs
- 60g walnuts

Directions
1. Clean the cauliflower by eliminating the green leaves and the central core, and always with the help of a smooth blade knife, detach all the tops, dividing in half the bigger ones. Transfer the cleaned buds into a colander and rinse them under cold water.
2. Situate saucepan full of water on the fire and as soon as it boils, dip the cauliflower tops, cooking them for about 10 minutes; the consistency will have to remain rather al dente, since it will be sautéed in the pan; then continue with the cooking in the oven. Drain the cauliflower into a bowl and leave it aside.
3. Heat a drizzle of oil in a large pan, add the onion and sauté over low heat. Once golden, add the cauliflower, salt, and pepper to taste. Stir and let everything season for about 5-6 minutes.
4. In the meantime, clean the red chicory by removing the central core, slice it thinly and mix to the pan with the cauliflower; stir, and fry for a few seconds so as not to wither too much.
5. Put out the fire and set aside. Chop the nuts.
6. Heat the oven to 200 °C in static mode. Grease 4 bowls with a diameter of about 11 cm and fill them with cauliflower and red chicory, sprinkle on the surface a pinch of breadcrumbs and walnut grains.
7. Bake for about 15 minutes, gratinating the last minutes of cooking with the grill to brown the surface. Remove from the oven and serve hot.

Nutrition: 429 calories 31g fats 27g protein

Red Chicory and Kale Salad

Preparation Time: 18 minutes
Cooking Time: 0 minutes
Serving: 4

Ingredients:
- 200 g of canned chickpeas
- 1 kale

- 1 red chicory
- 1 red onion
- 40g extra virgin olive oil
- Salt
- Lemon juice
- Walnuts
- Rocket salad

Directions
1. Clean the kale leaves and cut them into strips. Let them wither with finely chopped red onion in a non-stick pan with two tablespoons of extra virgin olive oil.
2. When the kale is cooked, mix it with the chickpeas, drained from their preserving liquid, in a salad bowl. The ingredient that will give that bitters' touch to the dish will be the red chicory, to be used raw.
3. Mix the various components and then season with fine salt, good extra virgin olive oil, and a splash of lemon, which will give acidity to the dish. Add the walnuts and some arugula leaves!

Nutrition: 427 calories 26g fat 14g protein

Egg Scramble with Kale
Preparation Time: 17 minutes
Cooking Time: 4 minutes
Serving: 3

Ingredients
- 4 eggs
- 1/8 teaspoon ground turmeric
- Salt and ground black pepper, to taste
- 1 tablespoon water
- 2 teaspoons olive oil
- 1 cup fresh kale, tough ribs removed and chopped

Direction
1. Beat eggs, turmeric, salt, black pepper, and water until foamy.
2. In a wok, heat the oil over medium heat.
3. Add the egg mixture and stir to combine.
4. Decrease heat to medium-low and cook for a minute.
5. Mix in the kale and cook for about 3–4 minutes, stirring frequently.
6. Remove from the heat and serve immediately.

Nutrition 183 Calories 13g Fat 12g Protein

Buckwheat Porridge
Preparation Time: 9 minutes
Cooking Time: 19 minutes
Servings: 2

Ingredients
- 1 cup buckwheat, rinsed
- 1 cup unsweetened almond milk
- 1 cup water
- ½ teaspoon ground cinnamon
- ½ teaspoon vanilla extract
- 1–2 tablespoons raw honey
- ¼ cup fresh blueberries

Direction
1. Mix all the ingredients (except blueberries and honey) on medium-high heat and boil.
2. Now, reduce the heat to low and simmer, covered for about 10 minutes.
3. Drizzle honey and remove from the heat.
4. Set aside, covered, for about 5 minutes.
5. With a fork, fluff the mixture, and transfer into serving bowls.
6. Top with blueberries and serve.

Nutrition 358 Calories 4.7g Fat 12g Protein

Eggs with Kale
Preparation Time: 13 minutes
Cooking Time: 28 minutes
Servings: 4

Ingredients
- 2 tablespoons olive oil
- 1 yellow onion, chopped
- 2 garlic cloves, minced
- 1 cup tomatoes, chopped
- ½ pound fresh kale, tough ribs removed and chopped
- 1 teaspoon ground cumin
- ¼ teaspoon red pepper flakes, crushed
- Salt and ground black pepper, to taste
- 4 eggs
- 2 tablespoons fresh parsley, chopped

Direction
1. Cook oil in a large wok over medium heat and sauté the onion for about 4–5 minutes.
2. Sauté garlic for a minute.
3. Add the tomatoes, spices, salt, and black pepper, and cook for about 2–3 minutes, stirring frequently.
4. Cook kale for 4 minutes.

5. Carefully, crack eggs on top of kale mixture.
6. With the lid, cover the wok and cook for about 10 minutes, or until desired doneness of eggs.
7. Serve hot with the garnishing of parsley.

Nutrition 175 Calories 11.7g Fat 8.2g Protein

SOUP AND STEW RECIPES

Miso Soup

Preparation Time: 11 minutes
Cooking time: 31 minutes
Serving: 3

Ingredients:
- 10 g wakame
- 1 liter of water
- 5 g (1 sachet) instant dashi granules
- 100 g tofu, chopped into cubes
- 1 heaping tablespoon (25 g) white miso paste
- 2 spring onions, cut and chopped

Direction
1. Place the wakame in a small bowl or cup and cover generously with water. Leave on for a few minutes.
2. Bring the 1-liter water to a boil in a large saucepan. Stir in the instant dashi powder until it has dissolved.
3. Turn down heat to simmer and stir the tofu. Add the wakame to the soup by discarding the water.
4. Let simmer for 2 minutes. Situate miso paste in a bowl and add a tablespoon of the dashi broth at a time.
5. Stir until the miso has dissolved and you have a smooth, thick sauce. Take the pan off the stove and stir in the miso. Try the soup and add a little more miso if desired.
6. Serve in two bowls and sprinkle the chopped green onion evenly over each dish.

Nutrition: 318 calories 24g fat 11g protein

Mexican Chicken Soup

Preparation Time: 13 minutes
Cooking time: 1 hour
Serving: 4

Ingredients:
- 4 chicken legs
- 2 shallots, peeled and roughly chopped
- 1 carrot, peeled and roughly chopped
- 1 liter of water
- 400 g of chopped tomatoes
- 300 ml passata
- 1 green pepper, deseeded and chopped
- 1 red chili, pitted and finely chopped
- 2 cloves of garlic, peeled and chopped
- 1 teaspoon dried mixed herbs
- 1 teaspoon paprika
- 1 teaspoon smoked paprika
- ½ teaspoon ground turmeric
- ½ teaspoon ground cumin
- 1 teaspoon mild chili powder
- 400 g canned black beans, drained
- 400 g canned kidney beans, drained
- 30 g (very large handful) parsley, chopped
- Salt and freshly ground black pepper

Direction
1. Place the chicken drumsticks, shallots, and carrots in a large saucepan. Pour over the water and bring to a boil.
2. Cook for 20 minutes, then remove the chicken drumsticks with a slotted spoon and set aside to cool.
3. Add the chopped tomatoes, passata, green pepper, chili and garlic and bring them back to boiling point.
4. Add the dried herbs, paprika, smoked paprika, turmeric, cumin and chili powder and simmer gently for 30 minutes.
5. Pull skin out from the chicken drumsticks and pull as much chicken off the bone as possible.
6. Cut the chicken and add it to the pan along with the black beans and kidney beans for the last 5 minutes.
7. Take out from heat and sprinkle parsley. Season generously.

Nutrition: 361 calories 35g fat 21g protein

Thai Spinach Soup

Preparation Time: 13 minutes
Cooking Time: 17 minutes
Serving: 4

Ingredients:
- 1 teaspoon olive oil
- 2 shallots, peeled and chopped
- ½ teaspoon ground cumin
- 1 thumb (5 cm) fresh ginger, peeled and grated
- 1 stick lemongrass

- 1 red chilies, deseeded, chopped
- Zest and juice of 1 lime
- 1 liter of boiling water
- 400 g coconut milk
- 250 g fresh spinach
- 1 tbsp Thai Green Curry Paste
- Large handful (20 g) parsley
- Large handful (20 g) of coriander

Direction:
1. In a large saucepan, cook olive oil slightly and fry the shallots for 5 minutes until they soften.
2. Add the cumin, fresh ginger, lemongrass, chili, and lime zest. Stir thoroughly, then pour in the water.
3. Bring to a boil, then add the coconut milk, simmer again slightly and cook for another 10 minutes.
4. Add the spinach and curry paste and simmer gently until the spinach is cooked through.
5. Remove from heat and throw away the lemongrass stick. Stir in parsley, coriander and lime juice.

Nutrition: 226 calories 21g protein 17g fat

Savoy Cabbage and Bacon Soup

Preparation Time: 12 minutes
Cooking Time: 37 minutes
Serving: 6
Ingredients:
- 200 g bacon or pancetta, roughly chopped
- 2 shallots, peeled and chopped
- 2 cloves of garlic, peeled and sliced
- 200 g white potatoes, peeled and roughly chopped
- 1.2 liters of boiling water
- 500 ml chicken broth, fresh or made with 1 cube
- 1 tsp English mustard
- 800 g savoy cabbage stalk removed and chopped
- 200 ml crème fraiche
- Large handful (30 g) parsley, roughly chopped

Direction:
1. Prep large saucepan over high heat and toss in the bacon. Fry for 3–5 minutes, turning regularly, until brown and crispy. Pull out with a slotted spoon and set aside. Add the shallots, stir and turn the heat on low.
2. Let the shallots cook for 5 minutes. Add the garlic and potato, sauté them for a few minutes then add the boiling water, chicken broth and mustard. Boil and simmer for 10 minutes. Stir the cabbage, return to the boil and cook for another 6 minutes.
3. Put in a blender in two batches and stir until smooth. Put the bacon back in and carefully heat the soup in the pan. Add the crème fraiche with a light fizz and cook for another 2 minutes before serving.

Nutrition: 296 calories 28g fat 16g protein

Edamame Beans Pesto Soup

Preparation Time: 13 minutes
Cooking Time: 41 minutes
Serving: 2
Ingredients:
- 1 teaspoon olive oil
- 1 leek, cut and sliced
- 1 clove of garlic, peeled and sliced
- 100 g white potatoes, peeled and diced
- 200 g fresh or frozen soy / edamame beans
- 3-4 basil leaves, torn
- 750 ml vegetable stock, fresh or prepared
- 50 g baby leaf spinach, shredded
- 1 tbsp pesto

Direction:
1. Cook oil in a large saucepan and gently fry the leek and garlic for 10 minutes. Add the potato, three quarters of the soybeans and the basil.
2. Boil broth, and simmer gently for 20 minutes. 2 Put the soup in a blender and stir until smooth. Situate soup to the pan and let it simmer gently. Stir in the remaining soybeans, spinach and pesto and heat for another 5 minutes.

Nutrition: 272 calories 26g protein 11g fat

Spicy Butternut Squash and Kale Soup

Preparation Time: 14 minutes
Cooking Time: 22 minutes
Serving: 4

Ingredients:
- 1 tbsp olive oil
- 2 shallots, peeled and chopped
- 1 clove of garlic, peeled and sliced
- 200 g sweet potato, peeled and diced
- 800 g (1 small) butternut squash, pitted, peeled and diced
- 1 red chili, pitted and chopped
- 1 teaspoon smoked paprika
- ½ teaspoon paprika
- 1 teaspoon ground turmeric
- 1 teaspoon salt
- 500 ml vegetable stock, fresh or prepared
- 1 liter of boiling water
- 1 tbsp whole grain mustard
- 20 g parmesan, finely grated
- 200 g of kale leaves, removed stems and roughly chopped
- 200 ml crème fraiche

Direction:
1. Cook oil in a large, thick-bottomed saucepan. Add shallots and garlic and stir-fry for 5 minutes.
2. Add the sweet potato and butternut squash. Stir, cover and cook gently for 10 minutes.
3. Stir in the chili, paprika, turmeric and salt. Boil stock and water. Let simmer for 20 minutes.
4. Put in a blender in two batches and stir until smooth. Return to the pan and gently heat it.
5. Add the mustard, parmesan and kale. Cook for 6 minutes. Add the crème fraiche, bring back to temperature and serve.

Nutrition: 234 calories 28g fat 11g protein

Kale Stilton Soup

Preparation Time: 13 minutes
Cooking Time: 31 minutes
Serving: 4

Ingredients:
- 1 tbsp olive oil
- 2 shallots, peeled and diced
- 2 leeks, cut and sliced
- 150 g white potatoes, peeled and diced
- 500 ml vegetable stock, fresh
- 500 ml of boiling water
- 400 g kale leaves, stems removed and roughly chopped
- 2 tbsp (30 ml)
- Sherry 200 ml skimmed milk
- 2 tbsp (30 ml) double cream (45% fat)
- 50 g Stilton, crumbled
- Large handful (20 g) parsley, roughly chopped
- Salt and freshly ground black pepper

Direction:
1. Cook oil in a large saucepan and gently fry the shallots and leeks for 10 minutes until tender.
2. Stir in the potato then add the stock and the boiling water. Boil, then reduce the heat and simmer lightly for 15 minutes.
3. Use a potato masher to mash the potatoes in the pan - or mix them in a blender if you prefer.
4. Add the kale, let it simmer gently, and cook for 4 minutes until the kale is just tender.
5. Add the sherry, milk, cream and half of the stilton.
6. Let simmer until the stilton has dissolved. Season generously with salt and pepper.
7. Divide into four bowls and serve with parsley sprinkled with Stilton.

Nutrition: 232 calories 24g fat 11g protein

Curry Broth

Preparation Time: 11 minutes
Cooking Time: 25 minutes
Serving: 4

Ingredients:
- 1 tbsp olive oil
- 2 shallots
- 1 clove of garlic
- 2 green chilies, pitted and finely chopped
- 1 teaspoon mild chili powder
- 1 teaspoon ground turmeric
- ¼ teaspoon cloves
- ¼ teaspoon ground cinnamon
- 1 teaspoon salt

- 150 g broccoli, cut into small florets
- 200 g kale leaves, stems removed and roughly chopped
- 400 ml chicken or vegetable stock, fresh
- 1 liter of boiling water
- 250 g tofu, cut into small cubes
- 2 spring onions, cut and chopped
- 20 g coriander, chopped

Direction:
1. Using large saucepan with a thick bottom, cook oil over low heat.
2. Add the shallots and sauté them for 5 minutes, until they just start to soften.
3. Add the garlic, green chilies, spices, and salt. Stir then add the broccoli and kale.
4. Fry for 2-3 minutes. Stir the stock and water and bring to a boil.
5. Let simmer gently for 15 minutes.
6. Add the tofu, spring onions, and coriander and cook for a few more minutes until it warms up.

Nutrition: 232 calories 23g fat 15g protein

Walnut Soup

Preparation Time: 16 minutes
Cooking Time: 1 hour
Serving: 1

Ingredients:
- 2 teaspoons of native olive oil
- 30g heard red onion
- 30 grams of heard celery
- 1 clove of heard garlic
- 1 teaspoon dried thyme
- 75 g canned or homemade white beans such as cannellini or haricot
- 500 ml vegetable broth
- 50 g kale, roughly chopped
- 4 chopped walnut halves

Direction:
1. Over medium saucepan, cook 1 teaspoon of olive oil over medium heat and fry the red onions, celery and garlic for 2-3 minutes. When soft, add the thyme, beans, and broth and bring to a boil.
2. Simmer at low heat for 25 minutes then stir the kale and cook for another 10 minutes. When all of the vegetables are cooked through, blend the mixture until smooth.
3. Prep your oven to 160 ° C / Gas 3 and roast your walnuts for 10-15 minutes. Serve with the remaining teaspoon of olive oil and topped with the roasted walnuts.

Nutrition 22g Fat 12g Protein 260 Calories

Spicy Lentils Vegetable Soup

Preparation Time: 13 minutes
Cooking Time: 31 minutes
Serving: 3

Ingredients:
- 1 teaspoon extra virgin olive oil plus
- 30 g red onion
- 30 g celery
- 30 g carrot
- 1 Birds Eye Chili
- 1 clove of garlic
- 1 teaspoon ground turmeric
- 1 tsp curry powder
- 500 ml vegetable broth
- 50 g red lentils
- 1 teaspoon chopped parsley

Direction:
1. With a small saucepan, heat the olive oil over low to medium heat and fry the onion, celery and carrot for 2-3 minutes until soft. Add the chili, garlic and spices and cook for another minute. Stir vegetable stock and lentils and bring to a boil. Simmer gently for 30 minutes and stir from time to time so that nothing sticks to the bottom.
2. Once the lentils have broken down and they have a nice soupy consistency, stir in the parsley and serve with a dash of extra virgin olive oil.

Nutrition 7g Fat 8g Protein 120 Calories

Watercress Soup

Preparation Time: 11 minutes
Cooking Time: 12 minutes
Serving: 2

Ingredients:
- 2 teaspoons of native olive oil
- 30 g of celery, smaller ties
- 30 g white onion, smaller rights
- 200 ml vegetable broth

- 50 g canned or homemade white beans such as cannellini or haricot
- 75 g watercress
- 1 tbsp chopped parsley

Direction:
1. Fill 1 teaspoon of olive oil in a small saucepan and cook the celery and onion gently for 2 minutes. Fill stock and beans, bring to a boil and cook over medium heat for 10 minutes.
2. Chop roughly the watercress and parsley, add to the pan and cook for 1 minute.
3. Remove from heat and stir until smooth. Serve the soup drizzled with the remaining teaspoon of olive oil.

Nutrition 11g Fat 5g Protein 130 Calories

Curry and Rice Stew

Preparation Time: 12 minutes
Cooking Time: 17 minutes
Serving: 4

Ingredients:
- 2 teaspoons of rapeseed oil
- 225 g paneer, cut into cubes
- Salt and freshly ground black pepper
- 1 red onion, sliced
- 1 thumb (5 cm) fresh ginger, peeled and grated
- 2 cloves of garlic, peeled and grated
- 2 fingers of chili peppers, heads removed and finely chopped
- ½ teaspoon aniseed
- 250 g cooked brown rice
- 250 g ready-to-eat or cooked Puy lentils
- 100 g frozen soy / edamame beans
- ½ teaspoon salt
- ½ teaspoon ground turmeric
- ½ teaspoon ground cumin
- ½ teaspoon ground coriander
- 1 teaspoon mild chili powder
- 2 tomatoes, chopped
- 50g baby spinach leaves
- Large handful (20g) parsley, chopped

Direction:
1. Cook oil in a large pan over high heat and add the paneer. Season generously with salt and pepper.
2. Cook the paneer, stirring frequently, until golden brown all over. Pull out and set aside.
3. Add the onion and reduce the heat in the pan to low. Before adding the ginger, garlic, chili peppers and anise, cook for 2 minutes and cook slowly for another 5 minutes.
4. Put the rice and lentils in a large bowl and mix gently, breaking up any lumps and separating the grains.
5. If the soybeans are frozen or need to be cooked, cook them according to the directions in the package. Add the salt, ground spices and chili powder to the pan and stir. Add the rice and lentil mixture, soybeans and tomatoes to the pan.
6. Stir very well and cook hot. Finally add the spinach and parsley and return the paneer to the pan.
7. Stir to combine and serve immediately. After cooling down completely, all spare servings can be chilled and served cold the next day.

Nutrition 19g Fat 24g Protein 347 Calories

Chinese Style with Pak Choi

Preparation Time: 17 minutes
Cooking Time: 1 hour
Serving: 4

Ingredients:
- 400 g firm tofu, cut into large cubes
- 1 tbsp corn flour
- 1 tbsp water
- 125 ml chicken stock
- 1 tbsp rice wine
- 1 tbsp tomato paste
- 1 teaspoon brown sugar
- 1 tbsp soy sauce
- 1 clove of garlic, peeled and chopped
- 1 thumb (5 cm) fresh ginger, peeled and grated
- 1 tbsp rapeseed oil 100 g shiitake mushrooms, sliced
- 1 shallot, peeled and sliced
- 200 g Pak choy
- 400 g minced pork (10% fat)
- 100 g sprouts
- Large handful (20 g) parsley, chopped

Direction:
1. Wrap tofu on kitchen paper, and set aside.
2. In a small bowl, mix the cornmeal and water and remove any lumps.
3. Add the chicken broth, rice wine, tomato paste, brown sugar and soy sauce.
4. Mix crushed garlic and ginger. Cook oil to a high temperature in a wok or large pan.
5. Add the shiitake mushrooms and sauté them for 2-3 minutes until cooked and shiny.
6. Take mushrooms from the pan with a slotted spoon and set aside.
7. Situate tofu in the pan and fry until golden brown on all sides.
8. Put the shallot and Pak choy in the wok, stir-fry for 2 minutes and then add the minced meat. Cook until cooked through, then add the sauce, reduce the heat by one notch, and let the sauce bubble around the meat for a minute or two.
9. Put the sprouts, shiitake mushrooms and tofu in the pan and warm through.
10. Take away from heat, sprinkle parsley and serve immediately.

Nutrition 19g Fat 36g Protein 347 Calories

Cauliflower Kale Curry

Preparation Time: 13 minutes
Cooking Time: 32 minutes
Serving: 4
Ingredients:
- 200 g buckwheat
- 2 tbsp ground turmeric
- 1 red onion, chopped
- 3 cloves of garlic, minced
- 2.5 cm piece of fresh ginger, chopped
- 1–2 chili peppers, chopped
- 1 tbsp coconut oil
- 1 tbsp mild curry powder
- 1 tbsp ground cumin
- 2 × 400 g cans of chopped tomatoes
- 300 ml vegetable broth
- 200 g kale, roughly chopped
- 300 g cauliflower, chopped
- 1 × 400 g can of butter beans, drained
- 2 tomatoes, cut into wedges
- 2 tbsp chopped coriander

Direction:
1. Cook the buckwheat following to the instructions on the package and add 1 tablespoon of turmeric to the water.
2. In the meantime, cook the onion, garlic, ginger and chili peppers in the coconut oil over medium heat for 2-3 minutes.
3. Add the seasonings, including the remaining tablespoon of turmeric and continue cooking over low to medium heat for 1–2 minutes.
4. Add the canned tomatoes and the broth and bring to a boil then simmer for 10 minutes.
5. Add the kale, cauliflower and butter beans and cook for 10 minutes.
6. Add the tomato wedges and coriander and cook for another minute.
7. Then serve them with the buckwheat.

Nutrition 17g Fat 8g Protein 270 Calories

Sirt Chicken Korma

Preparation Time: 16 minutes
Cooking Time: 51 minutes
Serving: 4
Ingredients:
- 350 ml chicken stock
- 30 g Medjool date, chopped
- 2 cinnamon sticks
- 4–5 cardamom pods, slightly split
- 250 ml coconut milk
- 8 boneless, skinless chicken thighs
- 1 tbsp ground turmeric
- 200 g buckwheat
- 150 ml of Greek yogurt
- 50 g of ground walnuts
- 2 tbsp chopped coriander

For the curry paste
- 1 large red onion, quartered
- 3 cloves of garlic
- 2 cm piece of fresh ginger
- 1 tbsp mild curry powder
- 1 teaspoon ground cumin
- 1 tbsp ground turmeric
- 1 tbsp coconut oil

Direction:
1. Situate ingredients for the curry paste in a food processor and flash for about a minute until you have a nice paste.

2. Fry the paste in a heavy pan over medium heat for 1-2 minutes then add the broth, date, cinnamon, cardamom pods, and coconut milk.
3. Bring to a boil then add the chicken legs. Reduce the heat, cover the pan with a lid, and simmer for 45 minutes.
4. Boil water and stir in the turmeric.
5. Add the buckwheat and cook according to the directions on the package. As soon as the chicken is tender, stir in the yogurt and cook the walnuts over low heat for a few more minutes.
6. Add the coriander and serve with the buckwheat.

Nutrition 16g Fat 32g Protein 330 Calories

Cauliflower Soup

Preparation Time: 12 minutes
Cooking Time: 47 minutes
Servings: 4

Ingredients:
- 3 pounds cauliflower, florets separated
- 1 yellow onion, chopped
- 1 tablespoon coconut oil
- Black pepper to the taste
- 2 garlic cloves, minced
- 2 carrots, chopped
- 2 cups beef stock
- 1 cup water
- ½ cup coconut milk
- 1 teaspoon olive oil
- 2 tablespoons parsley, chopped

Directions:
1. Heat a pot with the coconut oil over medium-high heat, add carrots, onion, and garlic, stir, and cook for 5 minutes.
2. Add cauliflower, water, and stock, stir, bring to a boil, cover, and cook for 45 minutes.
3. Transfer soup to your blender and pulse well, add coconut milk, pulse well again, ladle into bowls, drizzle the olive oil over the soup, sprinkle parsley and serve for lunch.

Nutrition: 190 Calories 2g Fat 4g Protein

Broccoli Soup

Preparation Time: 13 minutes
Cooking Time: 1 hour
Servings: 4

Ingredients:
- 2 pounds broccoli, florets separated
- 1 yellow onion, chopped
- 1 tablespoon olive oil
- Black pepper to the taste
- 1 cup celery, chopped   2 carrots, chopped
- 3 and ½ cups low-sodium chicken stock
- 1 tablespoon cilantro chopped

Directions:
1. Heat a pot with the oil over medium-high heat, add the onion, celery, and carrots, stir, and cook for 5 minutes. Add broccoli, black pepper, and stock, stir, and cook over medium heat for 1 hour.
2. Pulse using an immersion blender, add cilantro, stir the soup

Nutrition: 170 Calories 2g Fat 3g Fiber

Shrimp Soup

Preparation Time: 12 minutes
Cooking Time: 15 minutes
Servings: 6

Ingredients:
- 46 ounces low-sodium chicken stock
- 3 cups shrimp, peeled and deveined
- A pinch of black pepper
- 2 tablespoons green onions, chopped
- 1 teaspoon dill, chopped

Directions:
1. Put the stock in a pot, bring to a simmer over medium heat, add black pepper, onion, and shrimp, stir and simmer for 8-10 minutes.
2. Add dill, stir, cook for 5 minutes more, ladle into bowls and serve.

Nutrition: 190 Calories 7g Fat 8g Protein

Parmesan Tomato Soup

Preparation Time: 11 minutes
Cooking Time: 24 minutes
Servings: 4

Ingredients:
- ½ cup tomatoes, chopped
- 1 tablespoon tomato paste
- 1 teaspoon garlic, diced
- 2 cups beef broth
- 1 teaspoon chili pepper
- 2 oz Parmesan, grated

- 1/3 cup fresh cilantro, chopped
- 2 potatoes, chopped

Directions:
1. Mix up together tomatoes and tomato paste and transfer the mixture in the pan.
2. Add garlic and beef broth.
3. Add chopped potatoes and chili pepper.
4. Boil the ingredients for 15 minutes or until potato is soft.
5. Then blend the mixture with the help of the hand blender or in the food processor.
6. Add chopped cilantro and simmer the soup for 5 minutes.
7. Ladle the cooked soup in the serving bowls and top every bowl with Parmesan generously.

Nutrition: 148 Calories 3.9g Fat 9.2g Protein

Meatball Soup

Preparation Time: 13 minutes
Cooking Time: 28 minutes
Servings: 4

Ingredients:
- 1 cup ground beef
- 1 tablespoon semolina
- ½ teaspoon salt
- 1 egg yolk
- ½ teaspoon ground black pepper
- 4 cups chicken stock
- 1 carrot, chopped
- 1 yellow onion, diced
- 1 tablespoon butter
- ½ teaspoon turmeric
- ½ teaspoon garlic powder

Directions:
1. Toss butter in the skillet and heat it until it is melted.
2. Add onion and cook it until light brown.
3. Meanwhile, pour chicken stock in the pan.
4. Add garlic powder and turmeric.
5. Bring the liquid to boil. Add chopped carrot and boil it for 10 minutes.
6. In the mixing bowl, mix up together ground beef, semolina, salt, egg yolk, and ground black pepper.
7. Make the small sized meatballs.
8. Put the meatballs in the chicken stock.
9. Add cooked onion.
10. Cook the soup for 15 minutes over the medium-low heat.

Nutrition: 143 Calories 8.8g Fat 8.8g Protein

Eggplant Soup

Preparation Time: 12 minutes
Cooking Time: 31 minutes
Servings: 4

Ingredients:
- ½ cup tomatoes, chopped
- 2 eggplants, trimmed
- ¼ cup fresh parsley, chopped
- ¼ cup fresh cilantro, chopped
- 1 yellow onion, diced
- ½ teaspoon ground cumin
- ½ teaspoon cayenne pepper
- 1 celery stalk, chopped
- 1 tablespoon olive oil
- 1 teaspoon salt
- 1 garlic clove, peeled
- 1 teaspoon butter
- 4 cups chicken stock

Directions:
1. Peel eggplants and sprinkle them with olive oil and salt.
2. Preheat the oven to 360F.
3. Put the eggplants in the tray and transfer it in the preheated oven.
4. Bake the vegetables for 25 minutes.
5. Meanwhile, pour chicken stock in the pan.
6. Add chopped tomatoes, parsley, cilantro, ground cumin, cayenne pepper, celery stalk, and diced garlic clove.
7. Simmer the mixture for 5 minutes.
8. Meanwhile, heat the butter in the skillet.
9. Add onion and roast it until translucent.
10. Add the onion in the boiled chicken stock mixture.
11. When the eggplants are cooked, transfer them in the food processor and blend until smooth.
12. After this, put the blended eggplants in the chicken stock mixture.
13. Blend the soup until you get a creamy texture.
14. Simmer the soup for 5 minutes.

Nutrition: 137 Calories 5.7g Fat 4.2g Protein

Lemon Lamb Soup

Preparation Time: 12 minutes

Cooking Time: 51 minutes
Servings: 8

Ingredients:
- 1 ½-pound lamb bone in
- 4 eggs, beaten
- 2 cups lettuce, chopped
- 1 tablespoon chives, chopped
- ½ cup fresh dill, chopped
- ½ cup lemon juice
- 1 teaspoon salt
- ½ teaspoon white pepper
- 2 tablespoons avocado oil
- 5 cups of water

Directions:
1. Chop the lamb roughly and place in the pan.
2. Add avocado oil and roast the meat for 10 minutes over the medium heat. Stir it with the help of spatula from time to time.
3. Then sprinkle the meat with white pepper and salt. Fill water and bring the mixture to boil.
4. Scourge eggs and lemon juice.
5. Add a ½ cup of boiling water from the pan and whisk the egg mixture until smooth.
6. Add dill, chives, and lettuce in the soup. Stir well.
7. Cook the soup for 30 minutes over the medium-high heat.
8. Then add egg mixture and stir it fast to make the homogenous texture of the soup.
9. Cook it for 3 minutes more.

Nutrition: 360 Calories 22.9g Fat 33.6g Protein

Mushroom and Cheese Soup

Preparation Time: 14 minutes
Cooking Time: 18 minutes
Servings: 2

Ingredients:
- 1 cup cremini mushrooms, chopped
- 1 cup Cheddar cheese, shredded
- 2 cups of water
- ½ teaspoon salt
- 1 teaspoon dried thyme
- ½ teaspoon dried oregano
- 1 tablespoon fresh parsley, chopped
- 1 tablespoon olive oil
- 1 bell pepper, chopped

Directions:
1. Pour olive oil in the pan.
2. Add mushrooms and bell pepper. Roast the vegetables for 5 minutes over the medium heat.
3. Then sprinkle them with salt, thyme, and dried oregano.
4. Add parsley and water. Stir the soup well.
5. Cook the soup for 10 minutes.
6. After this, blend the soup until it is smooth and simmer it for 5 minutes more.
7. Stir in cheese until cheese is melted.
8. Ladle the cooked soup into the bowls. It is recommended to serve soup hot.

Nutrition: 320 Calories 26g Fat 15.7g Protein

Eggplant Stew

Preparation Time: 14 minutes
Cooking Time: 19 minutes
Servings: 4

Ingredients:
- ½ teaspoon cumin seeds
- 1 tablespoon coriander seeds
- ½ teaspoon mustard seeds
- 1 tablespoon olive oil
- 1 tablespoon ginger, grated
- 2 garlic cloves, minced
- 1 green chili pepper, chopped
- A pinch of cinnamon powder
- ½ teaspoon cardamom, ground
- ½ teaspoon turmeric powder
- 1 teaspoon lime juice
- 4 baby eggplants, cubed
- 1 cup low-sodium veggie stock
- 1 tablespoon cilantro, chopped

Directions:
1. Heat a pot with the oil over medium-high heat, add cumin, coriander, and mustard seeds, stir, and cook them for 5 minutes.
2. Add ginger, garlic, chili, cinnamon, cardamom, and turmeric, stir, and cook for 5 minutes more.
3. Add lime juice, eggplants, and stock, stir, cover, and cook over medium heat for 15 minutes. Add cilantro, stir, divide into bowls, and serve for lunch.

Nutrition: 270 Calories 4g Fat 9g Protein

Leeks Soup

Preparation Time: 12 minutes
Cooking Time: 75 minutes
Servings: 6
Ingredients:
- 2 gold potatoes, chopped
- 1 cup cauliflower florets
- Black pepper to the taste
- 5 leeks, chopped
- 4 garlic cloves, minced
- 1 yellow onion, chopped
- 3 tablespoons olive oil
- A handful parsley, chopped
- 4 cups low-sodium chicken stock

Directions:
1. Heat a pot with the oil over medium-high heat, add onion and garlic, stir, and cook for 5 minutes.
2. Add potatoes, cauliflower, black pepper, leeks, and stock, stir, bring to a simmer, cook over medium heat for 30 minutes, blend using an immersion blender, add parsley, stir, ladle into bowls, and serve.

Nutrition: 150 Calories 8g Fat 8g Protein

Pea Stew

Preparation Time: 19 minutes
Cooking Time: 23 minutes
Servings: 3
Ingredients:
- 1 carrot, cubed
- 1 yellow onion, chopped
- 1 and ½ tablespoons olive oil
- 1 celery stick, chopped
- 5 garlic cloves, minced
- 2 cups yellow peas
- 1 and ½ teaspoons cumin, ground
- 1 teaspoon sweet paprika
- ¼ teaspoon chili powder
- A pinch of black pepper
- ¼ teaspoon cinnamon powder
- ½ cup tomatoes, chopped
- Juice of ½ lemon
- 1-quart low-sodium veggie stock
- 1 tablespoon chives, chopped

Directions:
1. Heat a pot with the oil over medium heat, add carrots, onion, and celery, stir, and cook for 5-6 minutes.
2. Add garlic, peas, cumin, paprika, chili powder, pepper, cinnamon, tomatoes, lemon juice, peas, and stock, stir, bring to a simmer, cook over medium heat for 20 minutes, add chives, toss, divide into bowls and serve.

Nutrition: 272 Calories 6g Fat 9g Protein

Chicken Leek Soup

Preparation Time: 12 minutes
Cooking Time: 35 minutes
Servings: 4
Ingredients:
- 1 cup cabbage, shredded
- 6 oz leek, chopped
- ½ yellow onion, diced
- 1-pound chicken breast, skinless, boneless
- 1 tablespoon butter
- 1 teaspoon salt
- ½ teaspoon dried oregano
- ½ teaspoon dried thyme
- 1 tablespoon canola oil
- 4 cups of water

Directions:
1. Chop the chicken breast into the cubes and place in the pan.
2. Add butter and canola oil.
3. Cook the chicken for 5 minutes. Stir it from time to time.
4. After this, add yellow onion and chopped leek.
5. Add salt, dried oregano, and thyme. Mix up the ingredients well and sauté for 5 minutes.
6. Then add water and cabbage.
7. Close the lid and cook soup over the medium heat for 25 minutes.

Nutrition: 222 Calories 9.4g Fat 25g Protein

Carrot Soup

Preparation Time: 14 minutes
Cooking Time: 31 minutes
Servings: 6
Ingredients:
- 5 cups beef broth
- 4 carrots, peeled
- 1 teaspoon dried thyme

- ½ teaspoon ground cumin
- 1 teaspoon salt
- 1 ½ cup potatoes, chopped
- 1 tablespoon olive oil
- ½ teaspoon ground black pepper
- 1 tablespoon lemon juice
- 1/3 cup fresh parsley, chopped
- 1 chili pepper, chopped
- 1 tablespoon tomato paste
- 1 tablespoon sour cream

Directions:
1. Line the baking tray with baking paper.
2. Put sweet potatoes and carrot on the tray and sprinkle with olive oil and salt.
3. Bake the vegetables for 25 minutes at 365F.
4. Meanwhile, pour the beef broth in the pan and bring it to boil.
5. Add dried thyme, ground cumin, chopped chili pepper, and tomato paste.
6. When the vegetables are cooked, add them in the pan.
7. Boil the vegetables until they are soft.
8. Then blend the mixture with the help of the blender until smooth.
9. Simmer it for 2 minutes and add lemon juice. Stir well.
10. Then add sour cream and chopped parsley. Stir well.
11. Simmer the soup for 3 minutes more.

Nutrition: 123 Calories 4.1g Fat 5.3g Protein

Chickpeas Stew

Preparation Time: 13 minutes
Cooking Time: 41 minutes
Servings: 4

Ingredients:
- 1 teaspoon olive oil
- 1 cup chickpeas
- 4 garlic cloves, minced
- 1 yellow onion, chopped
- 1 green chili pepper, chopped
- 1 teaspoon coriander, ground
- ½ teaspoon cumin, ground
- ½ teaspoon sweet paprika
- 2 tomatoes, chopped
- 1 and ½ cups low-sodium veggie stock
- A pinch of black pepper
- 3 cups spinach leaves
- 1 tablespoon lemon juice

Directions:
1. Heat a pot with the oil over medium heat, add garlic, onion, and chili pepper, stir, and cook for 5 minutes.
2. Add coriander, cumin, paprika and black pepper, stir and cook for 5 minutes more.
3. Add chickpeas, tomatoes, stock, and lemon juice, stir, cover the pot, cook over medium heat for 25 minutes, add spinach, cook for 5 minutes more, divide into bowls, and serve.

Nutrition: 270 Calories 7g Fat 9g Protein

Green Beans Stew

Preparation Time: 13 minutes
Cooking Time: 22 minutes
Servings: 4

Ingredients:
- 2 tablespoons olive oil
- 2 carrots, chopped
- 1 yellow onion, chopped
- 20 ounces green beans
- 2 garlic cloves, minced
- 7 ounces canned tomatoes, chopped
- 5 cups low-sodium veggie stock
- 1 tablespoon parsley, chopped

Directions:
1. Heat a pot with the oil, over medium heat, add onion, stir, and cook for 5 minutes.
2. Add carrots, green beans, garlic, tomatoes, black pepper, and stock, stir, cover, and simmer over medium heat for 20 minutes.
3. Add parsley, divide into bowls, and serve for lunch.

Nutrition: 281 Calories 5g Fat 11g Protein

VEGAN RECIPES

Walnut Chocolate Cupcakes
Preparation Time: 9 minutes
Cooking Time: 40 minutes
Serving: 6
Ingredients:
- Buckwheat flour, 1 ½ cup
- Sugar, 2 cups
- Cocoa powder, 1 cup
- Salt, ½ tsp
- Almond milk, 1 ½ cup
- Vanilla extract, ½ tsp
- Coconut oil, ½ cup
- Walnuts, 2 tbsp
- Baking powder, 1 tsp

Direction:
1. Preheat your oven to 180 °C. Lay baking paper on the bottom of a cupcake pan.
2. Mix in flour, cocoa, and sugar and mix through. Mix in the vanilla extract, almond milk, coconut oil, walnuts, and baking powder and mix until it turns into a batter. Add boiling water and beat until it's evenly mixed in with the batter.
3. Pour in the batter evenly across cake cases, filling up to ¾ of each case. Bake for up to 18 minutes and let cool.
4. Optionally, you can add vegan icing.

Nutrition: 411 calories 21g fats 19g protein

Sirtfood Kale Smoothie
Preparation Time: 6 minutes
Cooking Time: 0 minutes
Serving: 1
Ingredients:
- Kale, finely chopped, 2 cups
- Raw honey, 2 tsp
- 1 banana
- 1 apple
- Fresh ginger, chopped, 1 tsp
- Half a glass of water, if needed

Direction:
1. Blend all the ingredients together and enjoy!

Nutrition: 107 calories 11g fats 6g protein

Fruity Matcha Smoothie
Preparation Time: 8 minutes
Cooking Time: 0 minutes
Serving: 2
Ingredients:
- Matcha powder, 2 tsp
- Milk, 1 ½ cup
- Raw honey, 2 tsp
- Melon, chopped, two cups
- Mint leaves, fresh, 2-3 pieces
- Lemon or lime juice, 1-2 tbsp

Direction:
1. Mix all the ingredients into a blender, starting from the liquids to melon, and top with milk, spices, and lemon/lime juice. Blend all together and enjoy!

Nutrition: 174 calories 17g fat 6g protein

Fresh SirtFruit Compote
Preparation Time: 19 minutes
Cooking Time: 0 minutes
Serving: 4
Ingredients:
- Green tea, fresh, ½ cup
- 1 lemon, halved
- 1 chopped apple
- Red grapes, seedless, 1 cup
- Strawberries, 2 cups
- Raw honey, 1 tsp

Directions:
1. Cook fresh green tea and 1 tsp of raw honey. Add the juice from ½ lemon and let cool.
2. Pour the grapes and strawberries into a bowl and pour the tea over the fruit. Serve after a couple of minutes.

Nutrition: 211 calories 14g fat 4g protein

Spicy Sirtfood Ricotta
Preparation Time: 11 minutes
Cooking Time: 34 minutes
Serving: 5
Ingredients:
- Extra virgin olive oil, 2 tsp
- Unsalted ricotta cheese, 200 g
- 1 chopped red onion
- 1 tsp of fresh ginger
- 1 finely sliced garlic clove
- 1 finely sliced green chili

- 1 cup diced cherry tomatoes
- ½ tsp ground cumin
- ½ tsp ground coriander
- ½ tsp mild chili powder
- Chopped parsley, ½ cup
- Fresh spinach leaves, 2 cups

Direction:
1. Heat olive oil in a lidded pan over high heat. Toss in the ricotta cheese, seasoning it with pepper and sea salt. Fry until it turns golden and removes from the pan.
2. Add the onion to the pan and reduce the heat. Fry the onion with chili, ginger, and garlic for around eight minutes and add the chopped tomatoes. Close lid and cook for another five minutes.
3. Add the remaining spices and sea salt to the cheese, put the cheese back into the pan and stir, adding spinach, coriander, and parsley. Cover and cook for 3 minutes.

Nutrition: 388 calories 27g fat 13g protein

Sirtfood Baked Potatoes

Preparation Time: 12 minutes
Cooking Time: 42 minutes
Serving: 8

Ingredients:
- Potatoes, 5 pieces
- Extra virgin olive oil, 2 tbsp
- Organic red wine, 1 tbsp
- 2 finely chopped red onions
- 4 finely chopped garlic cloves
- Finely chopped ginger, 1 tsp
- 1 chopped Bird's eye chili pepper
- Powdered cumin, 1 tbsp
- Ground turmeric, 1 tbsp
- Water, 1 tbsp
- Tomatoes, 2 small cans
- Cocoa powder, 2 tbsp
- Parsley, 2 tbsp
- A pinch of salt
- A pinch of pepper

Direction:
1. Ready oven to 200 °C. Bake potatoes for one hour. In the meantime, fry onions in olive oil for five minutes until they're soft. Add chili, garlic, cumin, and ginger and cook for another minute on low heat.
2. Add a tablespoon of water to prevent dryness. Mix in the tomato, chickpeas, pepper, and cocoa powder and let simmer for 45 minutes until the sauce becomes thick. Add parsley, salt, and pepper and serve with potatoes.

Nutrition: 391 calories 22g fat 14g protein

Spicy Quinoa with Kale

Preparation Time: 17 minutes
Cooking Time: 32 minutes
Serving: 4

Ingredients:
- Canned quinoa, 1 can
- Extra virgin olive oil, 1 tbsp
- 1 sliced red onion
- 3 finely chopped garlic cloves
- 1 finely chopped bird's eye chili
- Turmeric, 2 tsp
- Coconut milk, 2 cups
- Water, 1 cup
- Kale, chopped, 1 cup
- Buckwheat, 2 cups

Direction:
1. Fry the onions for five minutes in olive oil. Add ginger, garlic, and chili, and fry for another five minutes. Toss in the turmeric and wait for another minute. Then add in the quinoa and coconut milk, pour in a glass of water, and cook for 20 minutes. Cook kale for another five minutes.
2. Halfway through cooking the quinoa, fry the buckwheat in water for ten minutes. Drain and serve with the quinoa.

Nutrition: 401 calories 29g fat 17g protein

Mediterranean Sirtfood Quinoa

Preparation Time: 16 minutes
Cooking Time: 29 minutes
Serving: 5

Ingredients:
- Quinoa, 2 cups
- Extra virgin olive oil, 1 tbsp
- Finely chopped garlic cloves, 1 tbsp
- Fresh ginger, chopped, 1 tsp
- 1 sliced bird's eye chili
- 1 sliced red bell pepper
- Ground turmeric, ½ tsp

- Ground cumin, 1 tsp
- A pinch of salt
- A pinch of pepper
- Chopped kale, 1 cup
- Lemon juice, 2 tbsp

Direction:
1. Start off by cooking the quinoa. Pour into a pot, cover with two parts water, and bring to a boil. Let it boil for up to thirty minutes.
2. During the last five minutes, pan-fry the vegetables except kale in olive oil for up to five minutes. Once the vegetables have softened, add cumin, paprika, turmeric, salt, and pepper.
3. Stir through and insert quinoa. Stir again, add vegetable stock, and pan-fry until the excess liquid vapors out. Serve and enjoy!

Nutrition: 487 calories 31g fats 24g protein

Eggplant and Potatoes in Red Wine

Preparation Time: 8 minutes
Cooking Time: 43 minutes
Serving: 6
Ingredients:
- 1 large diced potato
- Finely chopped parsley, 2 tsp
- 1 sliced red onion
- Sliced kale, 1 cup
- 1 finely chopped garlic clove
- Sliced eggplant, 2 cups
- Vegetable stock, 1 ½ cup
- Tomato sauce, 1 tsp
- Extra virgin olive oil, 1 tbsp

Direction:
1. Preheat your oven to 220 °C.
2. Boil the potatoes for 6 minutes, strain, and roast in the oven for 45 minutes on 1 tsp of extra virgin olive oil. Turn potatoes over every ten minutes so that they cook evenly. Add chopped parsley once the potatoes are done.
3. Stir-fry the garlic, onions, and eggplant on olive oil for up to five minutes. Add the vegetable stock and tomato sauce, bring to a boil, and let simmer up to 15 minutes on low medium heat.
4. Serve with potatoes.

Nutrition: 491 calories 32g fats 16g protein

Potatoes with Onion Rings in Red Wine

Preparation Time: 11 minutes
Cooking Time: 32 minutes
Serving: 4
Ingredients:
- Diced potatoes, 3 cups
- Extra virgin olive oil, 1 tbsp
- Finely chopped parsley, ½ tbsp
- Red wine, 1 tbsp
- Vegetable stock, 150ml
- Tomato sauce, 1 tsp
- 1 sliced red onion
- Kale, sliced, 1 cup
- A pinch of salt
- A pinch of pepper
- 1 chopped bird's eye chili

Direction:
1. Boil the potatoes for up to five minutes and drain. Roast at 22o °C for 45 minutes. Add the parsley after taking the potatoes out of the oven.
2. Fry the onions for up to seven minutes in 1 tsp of olive oil and add kale and garlic. Add vegetable stock and let boil for up to two minutes. Serve alongside potatoes.

Nutrition: 341 calories 19g fats 8g protein

Sweet Potatoes with Grilled Tofu and Mushrooms

Preparation Time: 9 minutes
Cooking Time: 28 minutes
Serving: 4
Ingredients:
- Tofu, 14 oz
- Chicken stock, 1 cup
- Buckwheat flour, 1 tbsp
- Water, 1 tbsp
- Red wine, 1 tbsp
- Brown sugar, 1 tsp
- Tomato sauce, 1 tbsp
- Soy sauce, 1 tbsp
- 1 finely chopped garlic clove
- Ginger, finely chopped, 1 tsp
- Extra virgin olive oil, 1 tbsp
- Mushrooms, sliced, 1 cup

- 1 sliced red onion
- Kale, chopped, 2 cups
- Sweet potato, diced, 400 g
- Buckwheat, 1 cup
- Chopped parsley, 2 tbsp
- Vegetable stock, 2 cups

Direction:
1. Drain tofu by wrapping it in kitchen paper as you prepare other ingredients.
2. Cook buckwheat in vegetable stock. Add red wine, the tomato sauce, soy sauce, brown sugar, ginger, and garlic.
3. Stir-fry mushrooms for up to three minutes until cooked through. Add tofu and stir fry until the cheese turns golden. Remove from the pan and set aside.
4. Add the onions and stir fry for two minutes, upon which you'll add the diced sweet potatoes.
5. Pour more water or vegetable stock if needed, and add the sauce a minute or two before finishing. Combine the remaining ingredients and serve.

Nutrition: 361 calories 27g fat 18g protein

Buckwheat Stew

Preparation Time: 24 minutes
Cooking Time: 29 minutes
Serving: 5

Ingredients:
- 1 finely chopped red onion
- 1 finely chopped large carrot
- 1 finely chopped garlic clove
- Finely chopped celery, 3 tbsp
- Extra virgin olive oil, 1 tbsp
- 1 finely chopped garlic clove
- 1 finely chopped bird's eye chili
- Vegetable stock, 2 cups
- Rosemary, ½ tsp
- Basil, ½ tsp
- Dill, ½ tsp
- Celery, finely chopped, 1 tbsp
- Canned tomatoes, 400 g
- Buckwheat, 2 cups
- Kale, chopped, ½ cup
- Parsley, chopped, 1 tbsp

Direction:
1. Fry the onions, garlic, chili, celery, carrot, and spice herbs in olive oil on low heat. Once the onion turns soft, add the vegetable stock and tomato sauce.
2. Once the stock boils, add the buckwheat and let simmer for another half an hour. Add kale and parsley during the last five minutes.

Nutrition: 394 calories 24g fats 17g protein

Sirtfood Curry

Preparation Time: 13 minutes
Cooking Time: 27 minutes
Serving: 4

Ingredients:
- Skim milk
- Quinoa, 2 cups
- Chickpeas, 4 cups
- Potatoes, 14 oz
- Spinach, 1 ½ cup
- Tomato sauce, 1 tbsp
- 3 crushed garlic cloves
- Ground ginger, 1 tsp
- Ground turmeric, 3 tsp
- Ground coriander, 1 tsp
- Bird's eye chili powder, 1 tsp
- A pinch of salt
- A pinch of pepper

Direction:
1. Cook the potatoes for up to 30 minutes and drain. Move to a large pan and add all the ingredients except quinoa and bring to a boil.
2. Once the mixture has boiled, add the quinoa and chickpeas, and up to 1 ½ cup of water if needed. Decrease heat and simmer for 30 minutes while mixing regularly.

Nutrition: 374 calories 26g protein 14g fats

Onion Mushroom Salsa

Preparation Time: 9 minutes
Cooking Time: 14 minutes
Serving: 3

Ingredients:
- Mushrooms, 1 1/5 cups
- Ground turmeric, 2 tsp
- Lime juice, 1 tbsp
- Chopped Kale, 1 cup

- 1 sliced red onion
- Arugula, 1 cup
- Fresh ginger, chopped, 1 tsp

Direction:
1. Fry the mushrooms on a thin layer of extra virgin olive oil for up to five minutes, while stirring and making sure they're cooking evenly. As you fry, sprinkle turmeric over the mushrooms. Add kale half-way through, letting it soften only lightly. Prepare a plate and lay out fresh arugula.
2. Incorporate remaining ingredients together to make a salsa. Serve one dish next to another and enjoy!

Nutrition: 214 calories 1g fats 6g protein

Sirtfood Tofu Sesame Salad

Preparation Time: 14 minutes
Cooking Time: 4 minutes
Serving: 4

Ingredients:
- Sesame seeds, 1 tbsp
- 1 sliced cucumber
- Kale, chopped, 1 cup
- Arugula, 1 cup
- 1 fine sliced red onion
- Chopped parsley, ¼ cup
- Grilled tofu, diced, 2 cups
- Extra virgin olive oil, 2 tbsp
- Lime juice, 2 tbsp
- Soy sauce, 2 tbsp
- Raw honey, 1 tsp

Direction:
1. First, start by roasting sesame seeds for up to two minutes. Set aside to cool. If you've bought raw tofu, grill briefly on a thin layer of olive oil. Leave the remaining oil for salad dressing.
2. Mix vegetables and spices into a bowl. Toss in the chopped grilled tofu and sesame seeds, and mix to distribute evenly throughout the salad. To finish off, drizzle with lime juice and olive oil.

Nutrition: 451 calories 28g fat 14g protein

SALAD RECIPES

Cucumber Rolls on Cauliflower Salad

Preparation Time: 27 minutes
Cooking Time: 4 minutes
Serving: 4

Ingredients
- 600 g small cucumber (2 small cucumbers)
- 1 carrot
- ½ orange bell pepper
- 1 stick celery
- 1 avocado
- 2 tbsp sprouts
- salt
- pepper
- 1 cauliflower
- 50 g raisins
- 3 tbsp olive oil
- 3 tbsp lemon juice
- 1 ground cumin
- 1 pinch cinnamon
- chili flakes
- 4 stems parsley

Direction
1. Clean and wash the cucumbers and cut or cut lengthways into thin slices; cut the cut of the cucumber into narrow long strips.
2. Peel the carrot. Halve, core, and wash the peppers. Clean and wash the celery stick. Cut everything into thin finger-length strips.
3. Halve the avocado, remove the core, lift the pulp from the skin and cut into small slices. Wash the sprouts thoroughly and let them drain. Bundle some vegetable strips each and wrap them with a few sprouts in 1 cucumber slice, season with salt and pepper. Chill until served.
4. Clean, wash, and divide the cauliflower into small florets. Cook cauliflower in boiling salted water for about 5 minutes. Then drain, quench and let cool. Finely chop the cauliflower, mix with the raisins and oil. Season the cabbage with lemon juice, salt, pepper, cumin, cinnamon, and chili flakes.
5. Wash the parsley, shake dry and chop the leaves. Spread the cauliflower on a plate. Put 2–3 cucumber rolls and parsley on each.

Nutrition: 481 calories 26g fat 13g protein

Sweet Potato Salad with Spinach, Apple and Quinoa

Preparation Time: 23 minutes
Cooking Time: 14 minutes
Serving: 4

Ingredients
- 450 g large sweet potatoes (1 large sweet potato)
- salt
- pepper
- 1 map. curry powder
- 3 tbsp olive oil
- 200 g baby spinach
- 1 lemon
- 30 g walnut kernels (2 tbsp)
- 1 green apple
- 1 tsp maple syrup
- 2 tbsp vegetable broth
- 15 g puffed quinoa (4 tbsp)
- 5 g chive blossom (1 handful)

Direction
1. Skin sweet potato and cut it into bite-size pieces. Mix with salt, pepper, 1 pinch of curry and 1 tablespoon of oil and place on a baking sheet lined with baking paper.
2. Cook the sweet potato in a prep oven at 200 ° C (180 ° C fan oven; gas: setting 3), turning it bite-proof in 20 minutes, turning occasionally. Pullout and let cool for 10 minutes.
3. In the meantime, clean, wash and shake spinach dry. Drizzle lemon juice. Roughly chop walnuts. Clean, wash, quarter, core the apple, cut into small pieces and drizzle with half of the lemon juice.
4. Mix the remaining lemon juice with maple syrup, salt, pepper and remaining oil into a dressing.
5. Combine ingredients with the dressing in a bowl and divide into 4 bowls. Sprinkle the salad with quinoa and chive flowers.

Nutrition: 391 calories 26g fat 14g protein

Avocado and Mozzarella Salad Bowl

Preparation Time: 19 minutes
Cooking Time: 0 minutes
Serving: 4

Ingredients
- 60 g avocado
- Tomato 50 g
- Mozzarella cheese 40g
- Endive salad 20 g
- Raw lamb lettuce 10 g
- 2 tablespoons olive oil
- 1 fresh basil
- Sea salt 1 pinch
- Black pepper 1 pinch

Direction
1. Wash the lettuce leaves, drain well, then chop them into small bowls.
2. Wash and slice the tomatoes.
3. Slice mozzarella cheese. Wash the basil, shake to dry, and peel the leaves.
4. Remove the core by halving the avocado.
5. Take out avocado pulp from the skin and cut it into strips.
6. Add avocado, tomato, mozzarella, and basil to the salad.
7. Sprinkle with olive oil and season with a teaspoon of salt and pepper in a salad bowl.

Nutrition: 358 calories 21g fat 17g protein

Chicory and Orange Salad

Preparation Time: 39 minutes
Cooking Time: 0 minutes
Serving: 4

Ingredients
- 2 chicory
- 2 oranges
- 1 tsp honey
- 1 tbsp white balsamic vinegar
- 2 tablespoons of walnut oil
- Salt and pepper
- at will walnut kernels

Direction
1. Wash the chicory and cut into rough strips.
2. Fillets of 1.5 oranges, squeeze out the remaining half of the orange.
3. Mix the orange juice, honey, vinegar, oil, salt, and pepper well.
4. Add chicory and orange fillets and let steep for half an hour. Sprinkle with chopped walnut kernels as desired.

Nutrition: 314 calories 21g fats 14g protein

Mango and Avocado Salad with Watercress

Preparation Time: 14 minutes
Cooking Time: 0 minutes
Serving: 3

Ingredients
Salad:
- 3 handfuls of watercress
- 1 mango
- 1 avocado
- 1 spring onion
- 2 tbsp coriander leaves
- A little lime juices

Dressing:
- 2 cloves of garlic, finely diced
- 2/3 tsp ginger, finely diced
- 3 tbsp light sesame oil
- 1 tablespoon of rice vinegar
- Salt and pepper
- Some brown sugar
- 1 chili pepper without seeds
- a little dark sesame oil

Direction
Salad:
1. Clean, wash, spin dry watercress and cut it into bite-size pieces.
2. Peel the mango and avocado, remove the stones and cut the pulp into wedges. Immediately drizzle the avocado with a little lime juice so that it doesn't turn brown.
3. Rinse and slice spring onions into thin rings.
4. Pluck coriander leaves a little smaller depending on the size.

Dressing:
5. Sweat the garlic and ginger in half a tablespoon of heated light sesame oil, place in a bowl and let cool.
6. Mix in the vinegar, salt, pepper, and sugar.
7. Fold in the remaining light oil.
8. Add the chili to taste.

9. Season with the dark sesame oil.

Nutrition: 361 calories 28g fats 16g protein

Coconut Pancakes with Kiwi Salad

Preparation Time: 13 minutes
Cooking Time: 4 minutes
Serving: 4

Ingredients

Kiwi Salad
- 4 kiwi fruits
- 4 tbsp maple syrup
- 2 tbsp lemon juice

Pancakes
- 250 g flour
- 3 level teaspoons of baking powder
- 1.5 tablespoons of sugar
- salt
- 4 eggs
- 200 ml of coconut milk
- clarified butter

Direction

Kiwi Salad
1. Peel and dice the kiwi fruit. Then mix with the maple syrup and lemon juice.

Pancakes
2. Mix the flour, baking powder, sugar and 1 pinch of salt in a bowl.
3. Add the eggs and coconut milk and mix everything with the whisk to a smooth dough.
4. Heat a coated pan and melt approx. 1/2 tbsp clarified butter in it.
5. Put the dough in tablespoon-sized portions in the pan and bake for 4 minutes on each side.
6. Process the rest of the dough as well, adding a little clarified butter if necessary.
7. Serve the pancakes with the kiwi salad.

Nutrition: 391 calories 29g fats 12g protein

Salads with Oranges

Preparation Time: 13 minutes
Cooking Time: 0 minutes
Serving: 4

Ingredients
- 1 small red cabbage
- 2 teaspoons of salt
- 2 carrots
- 2 oranges
- 1 bunch of spring onions
- 1/2 bunch of parsley
- 3 tablespoons of balsamic vinegar
- 4 spoons of olive oil
- 1/2 tablespoon of mustard
- 1 pinch of Ceylon cinnamon powder
- black pepper, freshly ground
- 15 g of butter
- 2 spoons of honey
- 100 g of walnuts

Direction
1. Remove the wilted leaves from the red cabbage and cut it into quarters. Remove the stem.
2. Now cut the red cabbage into skinny strips or plan with the food processor.
3. Mix in a bowl with the salt and knead vigorously for 5 minutes so that everything mixes well.
4. Peel the oranges and peel off the white skin with a knife. Get the juice. Then cut the oranges into slices.
5. Mix vinegar, mustard, cinnamon, a little pepper, olive oil and orange juice and pour over the red cabbage. Let it go well.
6. Coarsely chop almost all the nuts, set aside only a few halves for decoration.
7. Heat the butter in a pan: first brown the decorative walnuts, then lightly brown the chopped walnuts. Chopped walnuts don't take long, so start with the halves.
8. Now add the honey to the nuts and mix well. Now immediately distribute the nuts on a plate and let them cool, otherwise they will join together.
9. Peel the carrots and coarsely grate them.
10. Squeeze the parsley and finely chop it.
11. Rinse spring onions and cut them into slices. Set aside some onions for decoration.

Nutrition: 341 calories 21g fats 18g protein

Autumn Salad

Preparation Time: 11 minutes
Cooking Time: 12 minutes
Serving: 4

Ingredients
- 150 g of corn salad
- 2 pears

- 60g of pink grapes
- 2 tbsp lemon juice
- 12 kernels of walnuts
- 2 spoons of honey
- 1 roll of goat cheese
- 2 spoons of butter
- 4 spoons of balsamic vinegar
- 6 spoons of water
- Salt and pepper from the mill
- 4 tablespoons of walnut or olive oil

Direction
1. Read the lamb's lettuce, clean, wash and spin dry.
2. The pear wash, cut into quarters and remove the seeds. Cut the quarters lengthways into narrow slits and immediately turn them into lemon juice.
3. Wash the grapes, pluck them from the stems, cut them in half and, if necessary, remove the stones.
4. Slice walnuts and roast them in a pan without fat until they smell slightly, then take them out.
5. Cut the goat cheese into finger-thick slices and grill briefly in the oven on a baking sheet (under baking paper).
6. Clean the pan and melt the butter in it. Sauté the pear slices in it, turning once. Add the honey and swirl everything well.
7. Deglaze with vinegar and water and bring to the boil briefly.
8. Remove from the heat, let the pear slices cool lukewarm in the brew, then remove from the brew.
9. Season the broth well, then stir in the oil vigorously.
10. Mix the lamb's lettuce in a bowl with the dressing and grapes, fold in the pear slices.
11. Sprinkle with walnuts and arrange the goat cheese on the plate.

Nutrition: 464 calories 31g fat 17g protein

Creamy Salmon Salad

Preparation Time: 16 minutes
Cooking Time: 32 minutes
Serving: 4

Ingredients
- 1 salmon fillet (130g)
- 40g mixed lettuce leaves
- 40g young spinach leaves
- 2 radishes, edged and thinly chopped
- Cucumber 5 cm (50 g), cut into pieces
- 2 spring onions, peeled and cut into slices
- 1 small handful (10 g) of parsley, coarsely chopped

For dressing:
- 1 teaspoon low-fat mayonnaise
- 1 tablespoon of natural yogurt
- 1 tablespoon rice vinegar
- 2 mint leaves, finely chopped
- Salt and freshly ground black pepper

Direction
1. Oven preheats to 200 ° C (180 ° C fan / Gas 6).
2. Situate salmon filet on a baking tray and bake for 18 minutes. Remove, and set aside from the oven. The salmon in the salad is equally lovely and hot or cold. If your salmon has skin, just cook the skin side down and remove the salmon from the skin after frying, using a slice of bread. When cooked, it should slide off easily.
3. Mix mayonnaise, yogurt, rice wine vinegar, mint leaves and salt and pepper then put aside for 7 minutes.
4. Situate the salad leaves and spinach with the radishes, cucumber, spring onions and parsley in a plate and top with salmon then sprinkle over the dressing.

Nutrition: 366 calories 27g fat 14g protein

May Beet Salad with Cucumber

Preparation Time: 19 minutes
Cooking Time: 10 minutes
Serving: 4

Ingredients
- 3 may turnips
- 1 cucumber
- 1 spring onion
- 2 stems parsley
- 150 g Greek yogurt
- 1 tbsp apple cider vinegar
- 1 tsp honey
- 1 tsp mustard
- sea-salt
- cayenne pepper

- pepper

Direction
1. Clean, peel and slice the turnips. Clean and wash the cucumber and also slicer. Rinse and cut the spring onions into rings. Put everything in a salad bowl and mix.
2. Wash parsley, shake dry and chop finely. Mix a dressing with yoghurt, apple cider vinegar, honey, mustard and 2–3 tbsp water. Season with salt and cayenne pepper.
3. Combine salad dressing with the mayonnaise and cucumber and let it steep for about 10 minutes, then grind it with pepper and serve.

Nutrition: 369 calories 19g fat 8g protein

Lentil Salad with Spinach, Rhubarb and Asparagus

Preparation Time: 14 minutes
Cooking Time: 0 minutes
Serving: 5

Ingredients
- 100 g beluga lentils
- 2 tbsp olive oil
- salt
- 250 g white asparagus
- 100 g rhubarb
- 1 tsp honey
- 50 g baby spinach (2 handfuls)
- 20 g pumpkin seeds

Direction
1. Bring the beluga lentils to the boil with three times the amount of water. Cook over medium heat for about 25 minutes. Drain, rinse and drain. Mix with 1 tablespoon of olive oil and a pinch of salt. In the meantime, wash, clean, peel and cut asparagus into pieces. Wash, clean and cut the rhubarb into pieces.
2. Heat 1 tablespoon of olive oil in a pan and fry the asparagus in it for about 8 minutes over medium heat, turning occasionally. Then add rhubarb and honey and fry and salt for another 5 minutes. Wash spinach and spin dry. Roughly chop the pumpkin seeds.
3. Arrange spinach with lentils, asparagus, and rhubarb on two plates and serve sprinkled with pumpkin seeds.

Nutrition: 381 calories 30g fat 16g protein

Spicy Onion Meatballs with Potato Salad

Preparation Time: 14 minutes
Cooking Time: 28 minutes
Serving: 4

Ingredients
- 400 g small potatoes
- 1 bunch radish
- 1 cucumber
- 1 bunch chives
- 2nd small onions
- 400 g beef steak or beef
- 1 egg
- 2 tbsp oatmeal
- 1 tbsp low-fat quark
- pepper
- salt
- 2 tsp rapeseed oil
- 250 ml classic vegetable broth
- 1 tbsp herbal vinegar

Direction
1. Wash the potatoes thoroughly, put them in a saucepan, cover with water and bring to a boil. Cover and cook for about 20 minutes.
2. In the meantime, wash, clean and slice radishes.
3. Peel and halve the cucumber with a peeler, halve the halves lengthways and remove the seeds with a spoon. Slice the cucumber.
4. Wash the chives, shake dry and cut the stalks into rolls.
5. Peel the onions and grate them in a bowl.
6. Add the mince, egg, oatmeal and quark. Season with pepper, knead well and form 4 meatballs with moistened hands.
7. Slowly fry brown on both sides in the hot oil in a coated pan over low heat. Heat the broth in a small saucepan.
8. Drain the potatoes, quench under cold water. Peel potatoes. It is best to impale it with a fork and remove the bowl with a small knife. Cut the potatoes into slices directly over a bowl and pour the hot broth over them.

9. Pour vinegar over the potatoes as well. Mix in the cucumber slices, radishes and chive rolls. Salt, pepper and serve with the meatballs.

Nutrition: 488 calories 34g fats 28g protein

Tomato and Zucchini Salad with Feta

Preparation Time: 13 minutes
Cooking Time: 0 minutes
Serving: 4

Ingredients

- 2 zucchinis
- 4 tbsp olive oil
- salt
- pepper
- 400 g tomatoes
- 200 g cherry tomatoes
- 3 spring onions
- 1 bunch basil (20 g)
- 2 tbsp apple cider vinegar
- 100 g feta (45% fat in dry matter)

Direction

1. Clean, wash, and cut zucchini. Heat 1 tablespoon of oil in a pan, fry the zucchini in it over medium heat for 5 minutes. Season with salt and pepper.
2. Clean, wash, and chop tomatoes. Wash and halve cherry tomatoes. Wash the spring onions and cut them into rings. Wash the basil, shake dry and pick the leaves.
3. Mix zucchini, tomatoes, cherry tomatoes, and basil. Add the remaining oil and apple cider vinegar, mix, and season with salt and pepper. Crumble the feta. Serve the salad sprinkled with feta.

Nutrition 355 calories 21g fat 13g protein

Cucumber and Radish Salad with Feta

Preparation Time: 13 minutes
Cooking Time: 0 minutes
Serving: 4

Ingredients

- 1½ cucumbers
- 1 bunch radish
- 1 bunch rocket (80 g)
- 4th gherkins
- 200 g feta
- 4 tbsp olive oil
- 3 tbsp lemon juice
- 1 tsp mustard
- 1 tsp honey
- salt
- pepper

Direction

1. Clean, wash, and cut cucumber and radishes into thin slices. Wash the rocket and shake it dry. Halve the pickled gherkins lengthways and cut into slices. Crumble the feta.
2. Whisk for the dressing oil with lemon juice, mustard, and honey, season with salt and pepper. Mix the cucumber, radish, and pickled cucumber slices and mix with the dressing. Place on a plate and sprinkle with the feta and rocket.

Nutrition: 264 calories 18g fat 8g protein

Baked Salmon Salad with Creamy Mint Dressing

Preparation Time: 16 minutes
Cooking Time: 28 minutes
Serving: 4

Ingredients

- 1 salmon fillet (130g)
- 40g mixed lettuce leaves
- 40g young spinach leaves
- 2 radishes, edged and thinly chopped
- Cucumber 5 cm (50 g), cut into pieces
- 2 spring onions, peeled and cut into slices
- 1 small handful (10 g) of parsley, coarsely chopped

For dressing:

- 1 teaspoon low-fat mayonnaise
- 1 tablespoon of natural yogurt
- 1 tablespoon rice vinegar
- 2 mint leaves, finely chopped
- Salt and freshly ground black pepper

Direction

1. Oven preheats to 200 ° C
2. Position salmon filet on a baking tray then bake for 16minutes. Pull it out, and keep aside from the oven.
3. Mix mayonnaise, mint leaves, yogurt, rice wine vinegar, and season well. Set aside for 5 minutes.

4. Arrange the salad leaves and spinach with the radishes, cucumber, spring onions and parsley. Situate salmon over the salad and drizzle the dressing.

Nutrition: 361 calories 22g fat 14g protein

Green Juice Salad

Preparation Time: 12 minutes
Cooking Time: 0 minutes
Servings: 1

Ingredients:
- 2 handfuls of chopped kale
- 1 handful of chopped arugulas
- 1 tablespoon chopped parsley
- 2 stalks of celery, sliced into bite-sized pieces
- ½ green apple, chopped into bite-sized pieces
- 6 walnuts, crushed
- 1 tablespoon olive oil
- ½ lemon, juiced
- 1 tsp grated ginger
- A pinch of salt and pepper

Directions:
1. Mix the juice of the lemon, ginger, seasonings, and olive oil into a small jar or small Tupperware container. Set aside until you are ready to eat.
2. In a large bowl or large Tupperware container, add your kale, arugula, parsley, celery, apple, and walnut. Mix it up until well combined and set aside until you are ready to eat.
3. When you are ready to eat it, shake up your dressing, then add it to the bowl and mix thoroughly.

Nutrition: 23g fat 12g protein 14 Calories

Strawberry Buckwheat Salad

Preparation Time: 21 minutes
Cooking time: 0 minutes
Servings: 2

Ingredients:
- 2/3 cup buckwheat
- 2 tablespoon turmeric powder
- 1 whole avocado, diced
- 1 whole tomato, diced
- ¼ cup diced red onion
- ¼ cup diced and pitted dates
- 2 tablespoon capers
- 1 ½ cups roughly chopped parsley
- 1 1/3 cups sliced strawberries
- Juice from 1 lemon
- Two cups of chopped arugula

Directions:
1. Cook your buckwheat with the turmeric powder added. Make sure that you follow the instructions that came on the package. When it is done, drain it and set it aside until it has completely cooled off
2. Mix all of your chopped ingredients together, keeping the arugula separate. Add the lemon and oil. Place all ingredients on top of the arugula and serve.

Nutrition: 122 Calories 13g Fat 9g Protein

Salmon Salad

Preparation Time: 23 minutes
Cooking Time: 0 minutes
Servings: 3

Ingredients:
- 3 cups of arugula
- 3 cups of chicory leaves
- ½ cup sliced smoked salmon
- ½ of an avocado, peeled and sliced
- 6 walnuts, crushed,
- 1 tablespoon capers
- 1 large Medjool date, pitted and chopped
- 1 tablespoon of olive oil
- ¼ lemon, juiced
- 10 sprigs of parsley, chopped
- 1 medium stalk of celery, chopped
- ½ cup thinly sliced red onion

Directions:
1. Chop and prepare all ingredients
2. Place salad leaves into a large bowl
3. Mix the remaining ingredients together in another bowl and pour on top of the leaves. Serve.

Nutrition: 188 Calories 26g Protein 6.2g fat

Chicken Sirtfood Salad

Preparation Time: 27 minutes
Cooking Time: 0 minutes
Servings: 1

Ingredients:
- ¼ cup plain Greek yogurt

- ¼ lemon, juiced
- 1 tsp cilantro, finely chopped
- 1 tsp turmeric powder
- ½ tsp curry powder (more to taste if you prefer it spicy)
- ¾ cup cooked chicken breast in bite-sized pieces
- 3 whole walnuts, crushed
- 1 Medjool date, pitted and diced
- 1/8 cup diced red onion
- 1 bird's eye chili, diced (remove seeds if you do not want it to be too spicy)
- cups roughly chopped arugula

Directions:
1. In a medium-sized bowl, combine your Greek yogurt, the juice from the lemon, your cilantro, and the curry and turmeric powders. Combine well.
2. Add in your chicken, walnuts, date, onion, and chili and mix together thoroughly.
3. Add to the top of the arugula. Serve.

Nutrition: 370 Calories 14g Protein 33g Fat

Sirtfood Pesto Buckwheat Salad

Preparation Time: 22 minutes
Cooking Time: 0 minutes
Servings: 4

Ingredients:
- 4 cups of parsley
- 1 tsp minced garlic
- 1 lemon, juiced
- ½ cup of walnuts
- 3 bird's eye chilies'—remove the seeds if you do not like spicy food
- ½ cup cauliflower, broken down
- 2 tablespoon parmesan cheese, freshly shredded
- 2 tablespoons extra virgin olive oil
- 2 tablespoon water
- Salt and pepper to taste
- 2 cups diced chicken breast, cooked
- 8 oz buckwheat pasta (dry weight), cooked

Directions:
1. Prepare your chicken and pasta, and set aside in a large bowl.
2. In a food processor, combine all ingredients aside from chicken and pasta. Blend until the consistency of pesto. Stop and scrape down walls from time to time to mix well.
3. Add 1 cup of pesto to the pasta and mix. If still dry, add more pesto to taste and mix well. Store in the fridge until ready to eat. This serves 4.

Nutrition: 379 calories 9.3g fat 4g protein

Kale Tofu Stir Fry

Preparation Time: 14 minutes
Cooking Time: 0 minutes

Ingredients:
For the tofu:
- 1 block of firm tofu
- 3 teaspoon curry powder
- 2 tablespoon soy sauce

For the stir fry:
- 3 large kale leaves, chopped
- 3 large arugula leaves, chopped
- ½ of a red cabbage
- 2 carrots, sliced
- 2 minced cloves of garlic
- 2 inches of minced ginger
- 4 tablespoon soy sauce
- 4 servings of buckwheat noodles

Directions:
1. Start by cutting up your tofu. It should be in bite-sized pieces. Then, mix in the soy sauce and the curry powder for the tofu and create a paste, which you will use to coat the tofu cubes. Set aside.
2. Cook your buckwheat noodles according to the package. Set aside when they are done.
3. Prepare all of your vegetables.
4. Prepare two frying pans with oil and turn them up to high. Put the tofu in one pan and cook until golden on all sides.
5. Add your garlic and ginger to the other pan and sauté for one minute
6. Add the kale, arugula, and cabbage to the garlic and ginger and cook until it begins to wilt. Then, add in the carrots and soy sauce. Cook for another two minutes.
7. Serve with pasta on the bottom, stir fry in the middle, and tofu on top, or store with pasta and stir fry in one container with the tofu in a separate one.

Nutrition: 232 Calories 8g Fat 10g Carbohydrate

Greek Stuffed Portobello Mushrooms

Preparation Time: 1 hour
Cooking Time: 42 minutes
Servings: 4

Ingredients:
- 3 tablespoons extra-virgin olive oil, divided
- ½ teaspoon ground pepper, divided
- 1 cup chopped spinach
- ½ cup quartered cherry tomatoes
- 1 clove garlic, minced
- ¼ teaspoon salt
- 2 tablespoons pitted and sliced Kalamata olives
- 4 Portobello mushrooms
- 1/3 cup crumbled feta cheese
- 1 tablespoon chopped fresh oregano

Directions:
1. Firstly, Preheat oven to 400 degrees F.
2. Mix 2 tablespoons oil, garlic, 1/4 teaspoon pepper and salt in a small bowl. Using a silicone brush, coat mushrooms all over with the oil mixture. Place on a large rimmed baking sheet and bake until the mushrooms are mostly soft, 8 to 10 minutes.
3. In the meantime, combine spinach, tomatoes, feta, olives, oregano and the remaining 1 tablespoon oil in a medium bowl. Once the mushrooms have softened, remove from the oven and fill with the spinach mixture. Bake until the tomatoes have wilted, about 10 minutes.

Nutrition: 345 Calories 54g Fat 6g Protein

Turmeric Sautéed Greens

Preparation Time: 3 minutes
Cooking Time: 0 minutes
Servings: 3

Ingredients:
- 1 tablespoon olive oil
- 1 2-inch piece fresh turmeric
- 1/4 teaspoon kosher salt
- 3 garlic cloves, minced
- 2 tablespoons water
- 2 bunches kale, spinach, or Swiss chard, thinly sliced

Directions:
1. Firstly, heat oil in a large sauce pan by using medium heat.
2. Now, add garlic and turmeric and sauté for 30 seconds.
3. Further, add kale and salt and sauté for 1 minute.
4. At the last add water to the pan and cook stirring until the greens are just wilted and serve.

Nutrition: 87 Calories 56g Protein 28g fat

Sautéed Collard Greens

Preparation Time: 21 minutes
Cooking Time: 17 minutes
Servings: 4

Ingredients:
- 1 slice thick-cut bacon, diced
- 1 bunch collard greens
- 2 garlic cloves, minced
- 1/2 teaspoon kosher salt

Directions:
1. Firstly, Put the bacon in a sauté pan over medium-low heat and cook for 5 minutes to render as much fat as possible.
2. While the bacon is cooking, remove the stems from the collard greens, and thinly slice the leaves across.
3. Now, add the garlic to the pan and cook for 1 minute. Add the greens and salt, stir well to coat the greens with the bacon fat, reduce heat to low, and cook for 5 minutes, until wilted, stirring occasionally. If you like them softer, cook for 10 minutes.

Nutrition: 87 Calories 10g Fat 56g Protein

Brussels Sprouts With Turmeric and Mustard Seeds

Preparation Time: 31 minutes
Cooking Time: 18 minutes
Servings: 2

Ingredients:
- 1 teaspoon oil
- 1/2 teaspoon (0.5 tsp) black mustard seeds
- 1/4 teaspoon (0.25 tsp) turmeric
- 3 cloves of garlic finely chopped
- 2 teaspoon or more sesame seeds
- 2 cups (176 g) Brussels sprouts
- 1/2 teaspoon (0.5 tsp) coriander powder

- 1 green chili finely chopped
- 1/2 teaspoon (0.5 tsp) cumin seeds
- 6 to 8 fresh or frozen curry leaves optional
- 1/2 teaspoon (0.5 tsp) garam masala optional
- cayenne to taste
- 1/2 teaspoon (0.5 tsp) salt or to taste
- 1/4 cup (62.5 ml) water
- cilantro and lemon for garnish

Directions:
1. First of all, heat oil in a large skillet over medium heat., When hot, put cumin and mustard seeds and cook until they change color or start to pop. Further, put curry leaves, garlic and chili carefully. Cook for a minute.
2. Now, add Brussels sprouts and toss well. Cook for 4 to 5 minutes until some edges get golden brown. Stir once or twice in between.
3. Put sesame seeds, mix in and cook for a minute. Mix in ground spices, salt and mix in and cook for a minute.
4. Add 1/4 cup or more water. Cover and cook for 7 to 9 minutes. This will steam the sprouts.
5. Finely, taste and adjust salt and heat. Add a dash of lemon and cilantro and serve.

Nutrition: 321 Calories 22g Fat 22g Protein

Sirt Salad

Preparation Time: 13 minutes
Cooking Time: 0 minutes
Servings: 1
Ingredients:
- 1 3/4 ounces (50g) arugula
- 1 3/4 ounces (50g) endive leaves
- 3 1/2 ounces (100g) smoked salmon cuts
- 1/2 cup (80g) avocado, stripped, stoned, and cut
- 1/2 cup (50g) celery including leaves, cut
- 1/8 cup (20g) red onion, cut
- 1/8 cups (15g) pecans, hacked
- 1 tablespoon tricks
- 1 huge Medjool date, hollowed and hacked
- 1 tablespoon additional virgin olive oil
- juice of 1/4 lemon
- 1/4 cup (10g) parsley, slashed

Directions:
1. Spot the serving of mixed greens leaves on a plate or in a huge bowl.
2. Combine all the rest of the fixings and serve on the leaves.

Nutrition: 108 Calories 33g Fat 44g Protein

Buckwheat Tabbouleh and Strawberry

Preparation Time: 43 minutes
Cooking Time: 23 minutes
Servings: 1
Ingredients:
- 1/3 cup (50g) buckwheat
- 1 tablespoon ground turmeric
- 1/2 cup (80g) avocado
- 3/8 cup (65g) tomato
- 1/8 cup (20g) red onion
- 1/8 cup (25g) Medjool dates, pitted
- 1 tablespoon escapades
- 3/4 cup (30g) parsley
- 2/3 cup (100g) strawberries, hulled
- 1 tablespoon additional virgin olive oil
- juice of 1/2 lemon
- 1-ounce (30g) arugula

Directions:
1. Cook the buckwheat with the turmeric as per the bundle directions.
2. Channel and put aside to cool.
3. Finely hack the avocado, tomato, red onion, dates, tricks, and parsley and blend in with the cool buckwheat.
4. Cut the strawberries and tenderly blend into the serving of mixed greens with the oil and lemon juice. Serve on a bed of arugula.

Nutrition: 234 Calories 3h Fat 6g Protein

Smoked-Tender Salmon Sirt Salad

Preparation Time: 24 minutes
Cooking Time: 0 minutes
Servings: 4
Ingredients:
- 1 cup, or ¼ package if large of smoked salmon slices
- 1 avocado, pitted, sliced, and scooped out
- 10 walnuts, chopped
- 5 lovage or celery leaves), chopped

- 2 celery stalks, chopped or sliced thinly
- ½ small red onion, sliced thinly
- 1 Medjool pitted date, chopped
- 1 tbsp. capers
- 1 tbsp. extra virgin olive oil
- 1/4 of a lemon, juiced
- 5 sprigs of parsley, chopped

Directions:
1. Wash and dry salad makings and vegetables, top with salmon.

Nutrition: 214 Calories 2g Protein 9g Fat

Coronation Chicken Salad
Preparation Time: 28 minutes
Cooking time: 0 minutes
Servings: 1

Ingredients:
- 75 g Natural yoghurt
- Juice of 1/4 of a lemon
- 1 tsp Coriander, chopped
- 1 tsp Ground turmeric
- 1/2 tsp Mild curry powder
- 100 g Cooked chicken breast, cut into bite-sized pieces
- 6 Walnut halves, finely chopped
- 1 Medjool date, finely chopped
- 20 g Red onion, diced
- 1 Bird's eye chili
- 2-ounce Rocket, to serve

Direction
1. Blend the yoghurt, lemon juice, coriander and spices together in a bowl. Add all the remaining Ingredients and serve on a bed of the rocket.

Nutrition: 122 Calories 13g Fat 9g Protein

Salad Buckwheat Pasta
Preparation Time: 26 minutes
Cooking Time: 22 minutes
Serving: 1

Ingredient
- 2 ounces of buckwheat pasta, cooked according to the directions for packaging
- Big pound of rye
- Tiny pound of basil leaves
- 8 Halved cherry tomatoes
- 1/2 Avocado
- 10 olives diced
- 1 Tablespoon of extra virgin olive oil
- 21/2 spoonful of pine nuts

Direction
1. Combine all the ingredients, except the pine nuts, gently and place them on a tray, then spread the nuts over the edges.

Nutrition: 322 Calories 17g Fat 8g Protein

Cucumber & Onion Salad
Preparation Time: 19 minutes
Cooking Time: 0 minutes
Servings: 2

Ingredients:
- 3 large cucumbers, sliced thinly
- ½ cup red onion, sliced
- 2 tablespoons olive oil
- 1 tablespoon fresh apple cider vinegar
- Sea salt, to taste
- ¼ cup fresh parsley, chopped

Directions:
1. In a salad bowl, place all the ingredients and toss to coat well. Serve immediately.

Nutrition: 81 Calories 5.8g Fat 1.3g Protein

Citrus Fruit Salad
Preparation Time: 16 minutes
Cooking Time: 0 minutes
Servings: 2

Ingredients:
For Salad:
- 3 cups fresh kale, tough ribs removed and torn
- 1 orange, peeled and segmented
- 1 grapefruit, peeled and segmented
- 2 tablespoons unsweetened dried cranberries

For Dressing:
- 2 tablespoons extra-virgin olive oil
- 2 tablespoons fresh orange juice
- 1 teaspoon Dijon mustard
- ½ teaspoon raw honey
- Salt and ground black pepper, as required

Directions:
1. For salad: in a salad bowl, place all ingredients and mix.
2. For dressing: place all ingredients in another bowl and beat until well combined.
3. Place dressing on top of salad and toss to coat well. Serve immediately.

Nutrition: 256 Calories 14.5g Fat 4.6g Protein

Mixed Berries Salad

Preparation Time: 17 minutes
Cooking Time: 0 Minutes
Servings: 4
Ingredients:
- 1 cup fresh strawberries
- ½ cup blackberries
- ½ cup blueberries
- ½ cup raspberries
- 6 cups arugula
- 2 tablespoons olive oil

Directions:
1. Toss all the ingredients to coat well.

Nutrition: 105 Calories 7.6g Fat 1.6g Protein

Orange and Beet Salad

Preparation Time: 18 minutes
Cooking Time: 0 minutes
Servings: 4
Ingredients:
- 3 large oranges, peeled, seeded and sectioned
- 2 beets, trimmed, peeled and sliced
- 6 cups fresh rocket
- ¼ cup walnuts, chopped
- 3 tablespoons olive oil
- Pinch of salt

Directions:
1. In a salad bowl, place all ingredients and gently, toss to coat.
2. Serve immediately.

Nutrition: 233 Calories 15.6g Fat 4.8g Protein

Strawberry, Apple & Arugula Salad

Preparation Time: 18 minutes
Cooking Time: 0 minutes
Servings: 4
Ingredients:
- 4 cups fresh baby arugula
- 2 apples, cored and sliced
- 1 cup fresh strawberries, hulled and sliced
- ¼ cup walnuts, chopped
- 4 tablespoons olive oil
- Salt and ground black pepper, as required

Directions:
1. For the salad, place all the ingredients in a large bowl and mix well.
2. For the dressing, place all the ingredients in a bowl and beat until well combined.
3. Pour the dressing over the salad and toss it all to coat well.
4. Serve immediately.

Nutrition: 243 Calories 19g Fat 2.9g Protein

Shrimp Salad

Preparation Time: 15 minutes
Cooking Time: 7 minutes
Servings: 6
Ingredients:
For Shrimp:
- 1 tablespoon olive oil
- 1 garlic clove, crushed
- 2 tablespoons fresh rosemary, chopped
- 1-pound raw shrimp, peeled and deveined
- ¼ teaspoon red pepper flakes, crushed
- Salt and ground black pepper, as required

For Salad:
- 8 cups fresh arugula
- 3 tablespoons olive oil
- 2 tablespoons fresh lime juice
- Salt and ground black pepper, as required

Directions:
1. In a large wok, heat oil over medium heat and sauté 1 garlic clove for about 1 minute. Add the shrimp with red pepper flakes, salt and black pepper and cook for about 4-5 minutes.
2. Remove the wok of shrimp from heat and set aside to cool. In a large bowl, add the shrimp, arugula, oil, lime juice, salt and black pepper and gently, toss to coat. Serve immediately.

Nutrition: 182 Calories 11g Fat 18g Protein

Smoked Salmon Sirt Salad

Preparation Time: 19 minutes
Cooking Time: 44 minutes
Servings: 3
Ingredients:
- 1 cup or ¼ package if large of smoked salmon slices no cooking needed!
- 1 avocado, pitted, sliced, and scooped out
- 10 walnuts, chopped
- 5 Lovage or celery leaves), chopped
- 2 celery stalks, chopped or sliced thinly
- ½ small red onion, sliced thinly

- 1 Medjool pitted date, chopped
- 1 tbsp. capers
- 1 tbsp. extra virgin olive oil
- 1/4 of a lemon, juiced
- 5 sprigs of parsley, chopped

Directions:
1. Wash and dry salad makings and vegetables, top with salmon.

Nutrition: 192 Calories 11g Fat 18g Protein

Waldorf Salad
Preparation Time: 12 minutes
Cooking Time: 0 minutes
Servings: 4

Ingredients:
- 250 gr of celeriac
- 250 gr of apples
- 70 gr of walnuts
- 150 gr of mayonnaise
- 200 gr of yogurt (thick)
- 1 tbsp. honey
- 1 lemon

Directions:
1. To prepare the Waldorf salad, start cleaning the celeriac, peel it by cutting the peel with a knife, wash it and cut it into slices and then into strips.
2. Bring the salted water to a boil and blanch the celeriac for 2-3 minutes, then drain and pat dry with a tea towel. Now move on to cleaning the apples, wash them, peel them and cut them into slices and then into strips.
3. Then dip the apples in water acidulated with lemon juice to prevent it from turning black (keep aside 1 tablespoon of lemon juice which you will need for dressing).
4. For the dressing, combine the mayonnaise, yogurt, a spoonful of lemon juice and honey, salt and pepper in a bowl, mix everything and add celery and apples.
5. Season the fruit and vegetables with the prepared dressing and add the coarsely chopped walnuts.

Nutrition: 243 Calories 20g Fat 2g Protein

Brown Rice Salad with Octopus
Preparation Time: 16 minutes
Cooking Time: 61 minutes
Servings: 6

Ingredients:
- 500 gr of octopus
- 250 gr of brown rice
- 2 courgette
- 1 clove of garlic
- 1 potato
- 1 egg

Directions:
1. First clean the octopus, then put it in a saucepan, cover it with cold water and put on the fire: cook for about 50 minutes after the boiling begins. Finally drain and let cool.
2. In the meantime, cook the rice, in abundant salted water, for the time indicated on the package, then drain it and let it cool too.
3. Cook the egg for 8 minutes from boiling to make it hard and boil the potato.
4. Wash and peel the courgette cut them into cubes and sauté them in a pan with a little oil and garlic. When they begin to soften, while remaining a little crunchy, add salt and pepper and let cool.
5. Cut the octopus into chunks, season it with salt, pepper, oil and parsley and add it to the courgette.
6. Also add the rice, the potato and the egg into chunks and gently mix everything.
7. Add potatoes and eggs.
8. Mix well.
9. Leave to rest in the fridge for 1 hour, and then serve your brown rice salad with octopus on the table.

Nutrition: 154 Calories 7.6g Fat 2.9g Protein

Exotic Rice Salad
Preparation Time: 8 minutes
Cooking Time: 21 minutes
Servings: 4

Ingredients:
- 250 gr of basmati rice
- 1 pineapple
- 200 gr of shrimp
- 150 gr of peas
- 50 gr of pecans
- 1/2 lime
- EVO oil

Directions:
1. Rinse the rice under running water several times until the water has become transparent.
2. Cook the basmati rice in a saucepan with plenty of salted water for the time reported in the package.
3. Once cooked, drain, and put the rice to cool
4. Cook basmati rice.
5. Sauté the shrimp and boiled peas in a pan with a spoonful of oil then cool prawns and peas.
6. Cut a pineapple in half lengthwise and empty it of the pulp, leaving in each half shell a border of a few millimeters.
7. Cut the flesh of the pineapple into cubes.
8. In a bowl put the rice; add the pineapple, peas and shrimp, season with the lime juice and a spoonful of oil.
9. Then add a handful of pecans and mix.
10. Put the exotic rice salad in the fridge for ½ hr. and serve.

Nutrition: 529 Calorie 10g Fat 9.5g Protein

Light Tuna and Bread Salad

Preparation Time: 17 minutes
Cooking Time: 8 minutes
Servings: 4

Ingredients:
- 4-5 slices of bread cut not too thin
- 3 boxes of natural tuna
- 4-5 not too ripe tomatoes for salad
- Salt and pepper
- 4 spoons of olive oil
- a pinch of oregano

Directions:
1. Heat a non-stick pan and in the meantime cut the slices of bread into coarse cubes. Add the bread to the pan, leaving it toasted well from all sides and then turning it often.
2. As soon as the bread is ready, let it cool.
3. In a salad bowl, or in four smaller bowls, put the bread, drain the tuna and distribute it on the bread, add a pinch of oregano.
4. We cut the tomatoes into not too regular cubes and put them in the salad.
5. At this point we can choose to season the salad with oil, salt and pepper and mix well, or use the condiments separately.

Nutrition: 180 Calories 10g Fat 11g Protein

Spicy Avocado Salad

Preparation Time: 7 minutes
Cooking Time: 0 minutes
Servings: 1

Ingredients:
- 1 avocado
- Few leaves of iceberg salad
- 2 green tomatoes
- Two tablespoons of mayonnaise
- Spoonful of ketchup
- Zest and juice of half a lime
- Small hot pepper
- Salt and pepper
- Extra virgin olive oil
- White vinegar a few drops

Directions:
1. Empty the avocado pulp and put it in a bowl by squeezing it
2. Add the green tomatoes cut into small cubes
3. Finely cut the chili pepper after removing the seeds
4. Cut the leaves of the iceberg salad into strips and add them to the rest
5. Put salt and pepper. Combine ketchup and mayonnaise, add the oil, the juice and the zest of the lime, the vinegar and mix everything
6. Use the avocado peel as a container.

Nutrition: 460 Calories 31g Fat 10g Protein

Hot Chicory & Nut Salad

Preparation Time: 8 minutes
Cooking Time: 42 minutes
Servings: 2

Ingredients:
For the salad:
- 100g 3½ oz. green beans
- 100g 3½ oz. red chicory
- 100g 3½ oz. celery, chopped
- 25g 1 oz. macadamia nuts, chopped
- 25g 1 oz. walnuts, chopped
- 25g 1 oz. plain peanuts, chopped
- 2 tomatoes, chopped

- 1 tablespoon olive oil

For the dressing:
- 2 tablespoons fresh parsley, finely chopped
- ½ teaspoon turmeric
- ½ teaspoon mustard
- 1 tablespoon olive oil
- 25mls 1fl oz. red wine vinegar

Directions:
1. Mix together the ingredients for the dressing then set them aside. Heat a tablespoon of olive oil in a frying pan then add the green beans, chicory and celery.
2. Cook until the vegetables have softened then add in the chopped tomatoes and cook for 2 minutes. Add the prepared dressing, and thoroughly coat all of the vegetables. Serve onto plates and sprinkle the mixture of nuts over the top. Eat immediately.

Nutrition: 438 calories 31g Fat 18g Protein

Tuna, Egg & Caper Salad

Preparation Time: 8 minutes
Cooking Time: 21 minutes
Servings: 2

Ingredients:
- 100g 3 ½ oz. red chicory or yellow if not available
- 150g 5 oz. tinned tuna flakes in brine, drained
- 100g 3 ½ oz. cucumber
- 25g 1 oz. rocket arugula
- 6 pitted black olives
- 2 hard-boiled eggs, peeled and quartered
- 2 tomatoes, chopped
- 2 tablespoons fresh parsley, chopped
- 1 red onion, chopped
- 1 stalk of celery
- 1 tablespoon capers
- 2 tablespoons garlic vinaigrette

Directions:
1. Place the tuna, cucumber, olives, tomatoes, onion, chicory, celery, and parsley and rocket arugula into a bowl. Pour in the vinaigrette and toss the salad in the dressing.
2. Serve onto plates and scatter the eggs and capers on top.

Nutrition: 340 calories 31g Fat 12g Protein

Nutty Fruit Granola

Preparation Time: 7 minutes
Cooking Time: 52 minutes
Servings: 2

Ingredients:
- 200g 7 oz. oats
- 250g 9 oz. buckwheat flakes
- 100g 3½ oz. walnuts, chopped
- 100g 3½ oz. almonds, chopped
- 100g 3½ oz. dried strawberries
- 1½ teaspoons ground ginger
- 1½ teaspoons ground cinnamon
- 120mls 4fl oz. olive oil
- 2 tablespoon honey

Directions:
1. Combine the oats, buckwheat flakes, nuts, ginger and cinnamon. In a saucepan, warm the oil and honey. Stir until the honey has melted.
2. Pour the warm oil into the dry ingredients and mix well. Lay out mixture out on a large baking tray then bake at 150C for 50 minutes. Allow it to cool. Add in the dried berries.

Nutrition: 220 Calories 2.5g Fat 6g Protein

DESSERT RECIPES

■ Snow-Flakes

Preparation Time: 9 minutes
Cooking Time: 8 minutes
Servings: 5
Ingredients:
- Won ton wrappers
- Oil to frying
- Powdered-sugar

Directions:
1. Cut won ton wrappers just like you'd a snow-flake
2. Heat oil when hot add won-ton, fry for approximately 30 seconds then reverse over.
3. Drain on a paper towel with powdered sugar.

Nutrition: 10g Carbohydrates 5g Fat 4g Protein

■ Lemon Ricotta Cookies with Lemon Glaze

Preparation Time: 12 minutes
Cooking Time: 19 minutes
Servings: 12
Ingredients:
- 2 1/2 cups all-purpose flour
- 1 tsp. baking powder
- 1 tsp. salt
- 1 tbsp. unsalted butter softened
- 2 cups of sugar
- 2 capsules
- 1 teaspoon (15-ounce) container whole-milk ricotta cheese
- 3 tbsp. lemon juice
- 1 lemon

Glaze:
- 1 1/2 cups powdered sugar
- 3 tbsp. lemon juice
- 1 lemon

Directions:
1. Pre heat the oven to 375 degrees F.
2. In a medium bowl combine the flour, baking powder, and salt. Set-aside.
3. Mix butter and the sugar levels. Using electric mixer beat the sugar and butter for minutes. Put eggs1 at a time, beating until incorporated.
4. Blend ricotta cheese, lemon juice and lemon zest. Stir in the dry skin.
5. Line two baking sheets with parchment paper. Spoon the dough on the baking sheets. Bake for fifteen minutes. Take it out and cool for 20 minutes.
6. Combine the powdered sugar lemon juice and lemon peel in a small bowl. Spoon 1/2-tsp on each cookie and flatten it. Allow glaze harden for approximately two hours. Pack the biscuits to a decorative jar.

Nutrition: 24.5g Carbohydrates 13.4g Protein 2g Fat

■ Homemade Marshmallow Fluff

Preparation Time: 7 minutes
Cooking Time: 17 minutes
Servings: 3
Ingredients:
- 3/4 cup sugar
- 1/2 cup light corn syrup
- 1/4 cup water
- 1/8 tbsp. salt
- 3 little egg whites egg whites
- 1/4 tsp. cream of tartar
- 1 teaspoon 1/2 tsp. vanilla infusion

Directions:
1. In a little pan, mix together sugar, corn syrup, salt and water. Attach a candy thermometer into the side of this pan, which makes sure it will not touch the underside of the pan. Set aside.
2. From the bowl of a stand mixer, combine egg whites and cream of tartar. Begin to whip on medium speed with the whisk attachment.
3. Meanwhile, turn burner on top and place the pan with the sugar mix onto heat. Allow mix into a boil and heat to 240 degrees, stirring periodically.
4. The aim is to find the egg whites whipped to soft peaks and also the sugar heated to 240 degrees at near the same moment. Simply stop stirring the egg whites once they hit soft peaks.

5. Once the sugar has already reached 240 amounts, turn noodle onto reduce. Insert a little quantity of the popular sugar mix and let it mix. Insert still another little sum of the sugar mix. Carry on adding and mixing slowly that means you never scramble the egg whites.
6. After all of the sugar was added into the egg whites, then turn the rate of this mixer and also keep overcoming concoction for around 79 minutes until the fluff remains glossy and stiff. In roughly the 5-minute mark, then add vanilla extract.
7. Use fluff immediately or store in an airtight container in the fridge for around two weeks.

Nutrition: 0.2g Carbohydrates 5g Fat 3.8g Protein

Banana Ice-Cream

Preparation Time: 6 minutes
Cooking Time: 11 minutes
Servings: 3
Ingredients:
- 3 quite ripe banana - peeled and rooted
- Couple of chocolate chips
- Two tbsp. skim milk

Directions:
1. Throw all ingredients into a food processor and blend until creamy.
2. Eat freeze and appreciate afterwards.

Nutrition: 0.3g Fat 23g Carbohydrates 3g Protein

Perfect Little Snack Balls

Preparation Time: 7 minutes
Cooking Time: 9 minutes
Servings: 4
Ingredients:
- 1/2 cup chunky peanut butter
- 3 tbsp. flax seeds
- 3 tbsp. wheat germ
- 1 tbsp. honey or agave
- 1/4 cup powder

Directions:
1. Blend dry ingredients and adding from the honey and peanut butter.
2. Mix well and roll into chunks and then conclude by rolling into wheat germ.

Nutrition: 3.1g fat 3.3g Carbohydrates 2g Protein

Loaded Chocolate Pretzel Cookies

Preparation Time: 7 minutes
Cooking Time: 14 minutes
Servings: 12
Ingredients:
- 1 cup yoghurt
- 1/2 tsp. baking soda
- 1/4 teaspoon salt
- 1/4 tsp. cinnamon
- 4 tbsp. butter softened
- 1/3 cup brown sugar
- 1 egg
- 1/2 tsp. vanilla
- 1/2 cup dark chocolate chips
- 1/2 cup pretzels tsp. chopped

Directions:
1. Pre heat oven to 350 degrees.
2. At a medium bowl whisk together the sugar, butter, vanilla and egg.
3. In another bowl stir together the flour, baking soda and salt.
4. Stir the bread mixture in using all the moist components, along with the chocolate chips and pretzels until just blended.
5. Drop a large spoonful of dough on an unlined baking sheet.
6. Bake for 15-17 minutes, or until the bottoms are somewhat all crispy
7. Allow to cool on a wire rack.

Nutrition: 40g Carbohydrates 8g Protein 288 Calories

Mascarpone Cheesecake with Almond Crust

Preparation Time: 12 minutes
Cooking Time: 21 minutes
Servings: 3
Ingredients:
Crust
- 1/2 cup slivered almonds
- 8 tsp. -- or 2/3 cup graham cracker crumbs
- 2 tbsp. sugar
- 1 tbsp. salted butter melted

Filling
- 1 (8-ounce) packages cream cheese, room temperature

- 1 (8-ounce) container mascarpone cheese, room temperature
- 3/4 cup sugar
- 1 tsp. fresh lemon juice (or imitation lemon-juice)
- 1 tsp. vanilla infusion
- 2 large eggs, room temperature

Directions:
1. For the crust: Set oven to 350 degrees. Blend almonds, cracker crumbs sugar in a food processor. Mix in butter.
2. Press the almond mixture on the base of the pan. Bake for 3 minutes. Cool. Decrease the oven temperature to 325 degrees f.
3. For your filling: with an electric mixer, beat the cream cheese, mascarpone cheese, and sugar. Stir in the lemon juice and vanilla. Add the eggs1 at a time, beating until combined after each addition.
4. Fill cheese mixture on the crust from the pan. Situate the pan into Pyrex dish fill enough hot water to the pan. Bake for 60 minutes. Transfer the cake to a stand for 1 hour. Refrigerate before cheesecake is cold, at least eight hours.
5. Use melted chocolate to decorate the cake!

Nutrition: 5g Carbohydrates 25g Fat 5g Protein

Marshmallow Popcorn Balls

Preparation Time: 7 minutes
Cooking time: 17 minutes
Servings: 12

Ingredients:
- 2 bags of microwave popcorn
- 1 12.6 ounces. Tote M&M's
- 3 cups honey roasted peanuts
- 1 pkg. 16 ounce. Massive marshmallows
- 1 cup butter, cubed

Directions:
1. In a bowl, blend the popcorn, peanuts and M&M's.
2. In a big pot, combine marshmallows and butter.
3. Cook medium-low warmth.
4. Insert popcorn mix, blend nicely
5. Spray muffin tins with nonstop cooking spray.
6. When cool enough to handle, spray hands together with non-stick cooking spray and then shape into chunks and put into the muffin tin to carry contour.
7. Add Popsicle stick into each chunk and then let cool.
8. Wrap each person in vinyl when chilled.

Nutrition: 1.1g Fat 3.2g Fiber 4g Protein

Homemade Ice-Cream Drumsticks

Preparation Time: 8 minutes
Cooking Time: 13 minutes
Serving: 4

Ingredients:
- Vanilla ice cream
- Two hazelnut chunks
- Magical shell - out chocolate
- Sugar levels
- Nuts

Directions:
1. Soften ice cream and mixing topping
2. Fill underside of sugar with magic and nuts shell and top with ice-cream.
3. Wrap parchment paper round cone and then fill cone over about 1.5 inches across the cap of the cone (the newspaper can help to carry its shape).
4. Shirt with magical nuts and shell.
5. Freeze for about 20 minutes, before ice cream is business.

Nutrition: 7g Fat 3g Protein 199 Calories

Ultimate Chocolate Chip Cookie Fudge Brownie Bar

Preparation Time: 11 minutes
Cooking Time: 13 minutes
Servings: 12

Ingredients:
- 1 cup (2 sticks) butter, softened
- 1 cup granulated sugar
- 3/4 cup light brown sugar
- Two big eggs
- 1 tablespoon pure vanilla extract
- Two 1/2 cups all-purpose flour
- 1 tsp. baking soda
- 1 tsp. lemon
- 2 cups (12 oz.) milk chocolate chips
- Inch kg double stuffed Oreos
- Inch family-size (9×1 3) brownie mixture
- 1/4 cup hot fudge topping

Directions:
1. Pre heat oven to 350 degrees f.
2. Cream the butter and sugars in a large bowl using an electric mixer at medium speed for 35 minutes.
3. Add the vanilla and eggs and mix well to thoroughly combine. In another bowl whisk together the flour, baking soda and salt, and slowly incorporate in the mixer till the bread is simply combined.
4. Stir in chocolate chips.
5. Spread the cookie dough at the bottom of a 9×1-3 baking dish that is wrapped with wax paper and then coated with cooking spray.
6. Shirt with a coating of Oreos. Mix together brownie mix, adding an optional 1/4 cup of hot fudge directly into the mixture.
7. Twist the brownie batter within the cookie-dough and Oreos.
8. Cover with foil and bake at 350 degrees f for half an hour.
9. Remove foil and continue baking for another 15 25 minutes.
10. Let cool before cutting on brownies might nevertheless be gooey at the midst while warm, but will also place up perfectly once chilled.

Nutrition: 7g Fat 25g Carbohydrates 3g Protein

Matcha Apple & Green Juice

Preparation Time: 13 minutes
Cooking Time: 0 minutes
Servings: 2
Ingredients:
- 5 ounces fresh kale
- 2 ounces fresh arugula
- ¼ cup fresh parsley
- 4 celery stalks
- 1 green apple, cored and chopped
- 1 (1-inch) piece fresh ginger, peeled
- 1 lemon, peeled
- ½ teaspoon Matcha green tea

Directions:
1. Mix all ingredients into a juicer and extract the juice following the manufacturer's method.
2. Split into two glasses and serve immediately.

Nutrition: 113 Calories 0.6g Fat 2.8g Protein

Apple, Cucumber & Celery Juice

Preparation Time: 14 minutes
Cooking Time: 0 minutes
Servings: 2
Ingredients:
- 3 large apples, cored and sliced
- 2 large cucumbers, sliced
- 4 celery stalks
- 1 (1-inch) piece fresh ginger, peeled
- 1 lemon, peeled

Directions:
1. Situate all ingredients into a juicer and extract it as per the manufacturer's method.
2. Divide into two glasses and serve.

Nutrition: 230 Calories 1.1g Total Fat 3.3g Protein

Lemony Apple & Kale Juice

Preparation Time: 11 minutes
Cooking Time: 0 minutes
Servings: 2
Ingredients:
- 2 large green apples, cored and sliced
- 4 cups fresh kale leaves
- 4 tablespoons fresh parsley leaves
- 1 tablespoon fresh ginger, peeled
- 1 lemon, peeled
- ½ cup of filtered water

Directions:
1. Place all ingredients in a blender and pulse until well combined.
2. Through a fine mesh strainer, strain the juice and transfer into two glasses.
3. Serve immediately.

Nutrition: 196 Calories 0.6g Fat 5.2g Protein

Watermelon Juice

Preparation Time: 7 minutes
Cooking Time: 0 minutes
Servings: 1
Ingredients:
- 20g of young kale leaves
- 250g of watermelon chunks
- 4 mint leaves
- ½ cucumber

Directions:

1. Remove the stalks from the kale and roughly chop it.
2. Peel the cucumber, if preferred, and then halve it and seed it.
3. Place all ingredients in a blender or juicer and process until you achieve a desired consistency. Serve immediately.

Nutrition: 0.6g Protein 7.6g Carbohydrates 0.2g Fat

Apple Muffins

Preparation Time: 13 minutes
Cooking Time: 14 minutes
Servings: 5
Ingredients:
- 2 eggs
- 1 cup oat flour
- ½ teaspoon salt
- 2 tablespoon stevia
- 3 apples, washed and peeled
- ½ cup skim milk
- 1 tablespoon olive oil
- ½ teaspoon baking soda
- 1 teaspoon apple cider vinegar

Directions:
1. Beat the eggs in the mixing bowl and whisk them well.
2. Add the skim milk, salt, baking soda, stevia, and apple cider vinegar.
3. Stir the mixture carefully. Grate the apples and add the grated mixture in the egg mixture.
4. Stir it carefully and add the oat flour.
5. Add the olive oil and blend into a smooth batter. Preheat the oven to 350 F.
6. Fill each muffin from halfway with the batter and place the muffins in the oven.
7. Cook the dish for 15 minutes.
8. Remove the cooked muffins from the oven.
9. Cool the cooked muffins well and serve them.

Nutrition: 200 Calories 6g Fat 11.7g Protein

Dark Chocolate Terrine

Preparation Time: 57 minutes
Cooking Time: 6 minutes
Servings: 10
Ingredients:
- For lubing the dish use vegetable oil
- 1/2 pound (2 sticks) unsalted spread
- 12 ounces ambivalent chocolate
- One teaspoon moment espresso powder
- 1 cup filtered confectioners' sugar
- 1/3 cup unsweetened cocoa powder
- Eight extra-huge egg yolks, at room temperature
- One tablespoon Cognac or liquor
- Touch of genuine salt
- Three extra-huge egg whites, at room temperature
- One tablespoon granulated sugar
- 1/2 cup cold overwhelming cream
- One teaspoon unadulterated vanilla concentrate
- Orange Sauce, formula follows
- Newly ground orange pizzazz, for serving
- Fleur de sel, for serving

Orange Sauce:
- Four extra-enormous egg yolks, at room temperature
- 1/2 cup sugar
- One teaspoon cornstarch
- 1 3/4 cups burnt entire milk
- One teaspoon unadulterated vanilla concentrate
- 1/2 teaspoons Cognac or liquor
- One tablespoon Grand Marnier alcohol
- 1/4 teaspoon ground orange pizzazz

Directions:
1. Softly oil an eight 1/2-by-4 1/2-by-2-inch portion skillet and line it as perfectly as conceivable with cling wrap, permitting the finishes to wrap over the sides. (I lay two bits of saran wrap transversely in the skillet, covering in the middle.) Place the container in the cooler.
2. Spot an enormous heatproof bowl over a dish of stewing water. Spot the margarine in the bowl, at that point the chocolate and espresso powder and warmth until simply softened, mixing once in a while with a flexible spatula. When the chocolate and margarine are dissolved, take the bowl off the warmth and speed in, each in turn, and all together, first the confectioners' sugar, at that point the cocoa powder, egg yolks,

Cognac and salt. Put the bowl in a safe spot for 15 minutes to cool.

3. Spot the egg whites and granulated sugar in the bowl of an electric blender fitted with the whisk connection and beat on fast until the white's structure firm however not dry pinnacles. Overlay the whites into the cooled chocolate blend with an elastic spatula.
4. Without cleaning the bowl or whisk connection, empty the cream and vanilla into the bowl and beat on fast until it frames firm pinnacles. Overlay the cream cautiously, however entirely into the chocolate blend. Fill the readied portion skillet, smooth the top, overlap the saran wrap over the top and chill for 4 hours or overnight.
5. To serve, turn the terrine out of shape and open it up. Spoon a puddle of Orange Sauce in every pastry plate and spot a cut of the terrine in the center. Sprinkle each serving delicately with orange pizzazz and fleur de sel.

For Orange Sauce:

6. Beat the egg yolks and sugar in the bowl of an electric blender fitted with the oar connection on medium-fast for 3 minutes, until exceptionally thick. Diminish to low speed and blend in the cornstarch.
7. With the blender still on low, gradually empty the hot milk into the egg blend (I utilize a fluid estimating cup for pouring). Empty the blend into a perfect, little, profound pot and cook over medium-low warmth, mixing continually with a wooden spoon, until it arrives at 180 degrees F on a treats thermometer and thickens to the consistency of overwhelming cream. The blend will cover the spoon. Try not to cook it over 180 degrees F, or the eggs will scramble! Promptly (it will continue cooking in the pan), pour the sauce through a fine-work sifter into a bowl, and mix in the vanilla, Cognac, Grand Marnier, and orange pizzazz. Spread and chill.

Nutrition: 175 Calories 7g Fat 3g Protein

Dark Chocolate Oatmeal

Preparation Time: 16 minutes
Cooking Time: 23 minutes
Servings: 4
Ingredients:
- 1/2 cups antiquated oats
- 1/4 cup unsweetened cocoa powder
- One teaspoon vanilla concentrate
- 1/2 teaspoon salt
- 1/3 cup nectar
- 1/2 cup cleaved toasted pecans
- Two bananas, cut into coins
- 1/2 cup dried fruits, plumped in warm water

Directions:
1. Heat 3 cups of water to the point of boiling in an enormous pot over medium warmth. Include the oats, cocoa powder, vanilla, and salt and cook, usually blending until thickened, 5 to 7 minutes. Mood killer the warmth and mix in the nectar. Spread and let represent 2 minutes.
2. Top each presenting with two tablespoons cleaved pecans, half of a cut banana and two tablespoons fruits. Serve right away.

Nutrition: 130 Calories 5g Fat 2g Protein

Dark Chocolate Nut Bars

Preparation Time: 75 minutes
Cooking Time: 22 minutes
Servings: 16
Ingredients:
- Two teaspoons virgin coconut oil
- 1 cup unsweetened coconut chips
- 1/2 cup hacked hazelnuts
- 1/2 cup hacked pecans
- 1/2 cup hacked cashews
- 1/2 cup trail blend (nuts as it were)
- One tablespoon ground flaxseed
- 1/2 cup maple syrup
- 1/3 cup nectar
- Legitimate salt
- 1/2 cup dull chocolate chips

Directions:
1. Special equipment: a candy thermometer
2. Preheat the broiler to 350 degrees F. Brush an 8-by-8-inch dish with one teaspoon of the coconut oil and put it in a safe spot.
3. Join the coconut chips, hazelnuts, pecans, cashews, trail blend, and flaxseed and spread into an even layer on a preparing

sheet. Toast until daintily brilliant, 10 to 12 minutes, at that point move to a large heatproof bowl. Put in a safe spot.
4. In a little pan, consolidate the maple syrup, nectar, and 1/2 teaspoon salt and heat to the point of boiling over medium-high warmth. Cook, sometimes mixing, until the temperature on a treat's thermometer peruses 260 degrees F, around 5 minutes. Promptly pour over the nut blend and mix to cover.
5. Utilize a flexible spatula to press the blend into the readied dish and let cool until set, around 30 minutes.
6. To make the chocolate sprinkle, consolidate the chocolate chips and staying one teaspoon coconut oil in a medium heatproof bowl and spot over a little pot of stewing water. Warmth, blending, until softened and smooth.
7. Shower the chocolate over the blend. At the point when set, cut into bars and serve.

Nutrition: 180 Calories 9g Fat 4g Protein

Dark Chocolate Martini

Preparation Time: 6 minutes
Cooking Time: 0 minutes
Servings: 1
Ingredients:
- Sugar
- Cleaved dull chocolate
- Vodka
- Coffee
- Orange

Directions:
1. Blend 2 tablespoons every raw sugar and finely cleaved dull chocolate on a plate. Consolidate 2 ounces every chocolate alcohol and vodka, 1-ounce chilled coffee, 1/2 teaspoon new squeezed orange, and a piece of orange get-up-and-go in a mixed drink shaker with ice; mix well.
2. Saturate the edge of a chilled martini glass and plunge it in the sugar-chocolate blend. Strain the mixed drink into the glass and trimmed with an orange wedge.

Nutrition: 405 Calories 39g Carbohydrates 8g Protein

Dark Chocolate Brownies

Preparation Time: 27 minutes
Cooking Time: 23 minutes
Servings: 24
Ingredients:
- 8 ounces ambivalent chocolate, coarsely cleaved
- Two tablespoons unsalted spread
- 1 cup entire grain cake flour*
- 1/4 cup unsweetened ordinary cocoa powder
- 1/4 teaspoon salt
- 1/4 teaspoon preparing pop
- Four huge eggs
- 1 cup stuffed light earthy colored sugar
- 1/2 cup plain low-fat yogurt
- 1/4 cup canola oil
- Two teaspoons vanilla concentrate
- 3/4 cup hacked pecans (discretionary)

Directions:
1. Preheat the stove to 350 degrees. Coat a 9 x 13inch preparing dish with cooking shower.
2. Dissolve the chocolate and spread in a twofold evaporator or heatproof bowl set over a pot of scarcely stewing water, blending every so often.
3. In a medium bowl, whisk together the flour, cocoa, salt, and preparing pop.
4. In an enormous bowl, whisk the eggs and sugar until smooth. Include the yogurt, oil, and vanilla, and race to consolidate.
5. Include the chocolate-spread blend and rush until mixed. Include the flour blend and blend until just soaked.
6. Move the blend to the readied container and sprinkle with nuts if utilizing. Heat for 20-25 minutes, until a wooden toothpick embedded in the middle comes out with a couple of sodden pieces. Cool totally in the skillet on a wire rack. Cut into 24 squares.

Nutrition: 140 Calories 3g Fat 2g Protein

Dark-Choco Mousse

Preparation Time: 22 minutes
Cooking Time: 1 hour
Servings: 5
Ingredients:
- 1 (12.3-ounce) bundle luxurious tofu, depleted

- 3 ounces great mixed chocolate, finely cleaved
- 1/4 cup unsweetened cocoa powder, ideally Dutch-prepared
- 1/4 cup water
- One tablespoon liquor
- 1/2 cup in addition to 1/2 teaspoon superfine sugar
- 1/4 cup substantial cream
- 1/4 teaspoons shaved chocolate

Directions:
1. In a blender or food processor, puree the tofu until it is smooth.
2. Put the slashed chocolate, cocoa powder, 1/4 cup water, and liquor in a pot or warmth proof bowl fitted over a pot containing 1-inch scarcely stewing water. Mix now and again, until liquefied and smooth. Expel from heat. Blend in 1/2 cup of sugar, a little at once, until smooth.
3. Add the chocolate blend to the tofu and puree until smooth and all-around mixed. Spoon the mousse into serving dishes, cover, and refrigerate for at any rate 60 minutes.
4. Whip the cream with a mixer. At the point when the cream is whipped, include the staying 1/2 teaspoon of sugar and get done with whipping.
5. Top each presenting with a bit of whipped cream and a sprinkle of chocolate shavings and serve.

Nutrition: 100 Calories 0.1g Fat 3g Protein

Strawberry Buckwheat Pancakes

Preparation Time: 7 minutes
Cooking Time: 42 minutes
Servings: 2

Ingredients:
- 100g 3½oz strawberries, chopped
- 100g 3½ oz. buckwheat flour
- 1 egg
- 250mls 8fl oz. milk
- 1 teaspoon olive oil
- 1 teaspoon olive oil for frying
- Freshly squeezed juice of 1 orange

Directions:
1. Pour the milk. Mix in the egg and olive oil. Sift in the flour to the liquid mixture. Heat a little oil in a pan and pour in a quarter of the mixture or to the size you prefer.
2. Sprinkle in a quarter of the strawberries into the batter. Cook for around 2 minutes on each side. Serve hot with a drizzle of orange juice.

Nutrition: 175 Calories 35g Fat 21g Protein

Strawberry & Nut Granola

Preparation Time: 7 minutes
Cooking Time: 51 minutes
Servings: 2

Ingredients:
- 200g 7oz oats
- 250g 9oz buckwheat flakes
- 100g 3½ oz. walnuts, chopped
- 100g 3½ oz. almonds, chopped
- 100g 3½ oz. dried strawberries
- 1½ teaspoons ground ginger
- 1½ teaspoons ground cinnamon
- 120mls 4fl oz. olive oil
- 2 tablespoon honey

Directions:
1. Combine the oats, buckwheat flakes, nuts, ginger and cinnamon.
2. In a saucepan, warm the oil and honey. Stir until the honey has melted.
3. Pour the warm oil into the dry ingredients and mix well.
4. Fill mixture out on a big baking tray and bake at 300F until the granola is golden.
5. Allow it to cool. Add in the dried berries. Store in an airtight container until ready to use.

Nutrition: 360 Calories 28g Fat 19g Protein

Chilled Strawberry & Walnut Porridge

Preparation Time: 8 minutes
Cooking Time: 53 minutes
Servings: 2

Ingredients:
- 100g 3½ oz. strawberries
- 50g 2oz rolled oats
- 4 walnut halves, chopped
- 1 teaspoon chia seeds
- 200 ml 7fl oz. unsweetened soya milk

- 100 ml 3½ fl. oz. water

Directions:
1. Place the strawberries, oats, soya milk and water into a blender and process until smooth. Stir in the chia seeds and mix well. Chill in the fridge overnight and serve.

Nutrition: 268 Calories 31g Fat 21g Protein

Sweet Oatmeal
Preparation Time: 8 minutes
Cooking Time: 11 minutes
Servings: 3

Ingredients:
- 1 cup oatmeal
- 5 apricots
- 1 tablespoon honey
- 1 cup coconut milk, unsweetened
- 1 teaspoon cashew butter
- ¼ teaspoon salt
- ½ cup of water

Directions:
1. Combine the coconut milk and oatmeal together in the saucepan and stir the mixture.
2. Add the water and stir it again. Sprinkle the mixture with the salt and close the lid.
3. Cook the oatmeal on medium heat for 10 minutes.
4. Meanwhile, chop the apricots into tiny pieces and combine the chopped fruit with the honey. When the oatmeal is cooked, add cashew butter and fruit mixture. Stir and serve.

Nutrition: 336 Calories 21.2g Fat 6.2g Protein

Watergate Salad Recipe
Preparation Time: 62 minutes
Cooking time: 0
Servings: 1

Ingredients:
- 2 (8-ounce) jars squashed pineapple in juice, undrained
- 1 (3.4-ounce) bundle pistachio moment pudding
- 1 (8-ounce) tub solidified whipped beating, defrosted
- 1 cup smaller than usual marshmallows
- 1/2 cup toasted walnuts, hacked

Directions:
1. In a medium bowl, mix together the full substance of the pineapple jars and the pudding blend until smooth.
2. Overlay in whipped fixing and marshmallows. Cover and refrigerate in any event 60 minutes. Sprinkle walnuts on top before serving.

Nutrition: 150 Calories 2g Fat 7g Carbohydrates

Moroccan Leeks Snack
Preparation Time: 13 minutes
Cooking time: 0 minute
Serving: 4

Ingredients:
- 1 bunch radish, sliced
- 3 cups leeks, chopped
- 1 ½ cups olives, pitted and sliced
- Pinch turmeric powder
- 2 tablespoons essential olive oil
- 1 cup cilantro, chopped

Directions:
1. Take a bowl and mix in radishes, leeks, olives and cilantro.
2. Mix well.
3. Season with pepper, oil, turmeric and toss well.
4. Serve and enjoy!

Nutrition: 130 Calories 4g Protein 3g Fats

Strawberry Pretzel Salad
Preparation Time: 46 minutes
Cooking time: 11 minutes
Servings: 4

Ingredients:
Pretzel Crust
- 3 1/2 cups pretzels, squashed
- 1/4 cup sugar
- 1/2 cup unsalted spread, dissolved

Cream Cheese Filling
- 8 Oz cream cheddar, mellowed
- 1/2 cup sugar
- 8 Oz cool whip, or whipped cream (solidly whipped)
- Strawberry Jell-O Topping
- 1 lbs. new strawberries, hulled and cut
- 2 cups bubbling water
- 6 Oz strawberry jelly powder

Directions:
1. Preheat stove to 350°F. Put aside a 9x13 inch glass preparing dish. Spot pretzels in a

Ziplock sack, seal and pound with a moving pin to smash daintily. In a medium bowl, mix together the liquefied margarine and sugar.
2. Include the squashed pretzels and blend to cover. Press the pretzel blend into the preparing dish, and afterward heat for 10 minutes. Expel from broiler. In a medium bowl, consolidate jelly powder with bubbling water.
3. Mix gradually for one moment until broke down and put in a safe spot. In a huge bowl, beat the cream cheddar and sugar until soft. Utilizing a huge spatula, crease in the cool whip until equitably mixed.
4. When the prepared pretzels are cool, spread the cream cheddar blend equitably on top until level over the dish. At that point, chill for at any rate 30 minutes. While chilling, you can wash, body and cut the strawberries.
5. Tenderly spot the cut strawberries onto the filling in a solitary layer. Include any residual strawberries top as a fractional second layer. When the Jell-O blend is room temperature, spill over the strawberries utilizing the rear of a spoon for even dispersion. Chill for in any event two hours. Serve and appreciate it!

Nutrition: 200 Calories 9g Carbohydrates 2g Fats

Sheet Pan Apple Pie Bake

Preparation Time: 22 minutes
Cooking Time: 16 minutes
Servings: 1

Ingredients:
- 8 flour tortillas, 8 inches
- 4 tbsp unsalted spread
- 8 Granny Smith apples, stripped, cored and cleaved
- 3/4 cup sugar, partitioned
- 3 tsp cinnamon, partitioned
- 1 tbsp lemon juice, new pressed
- Serving thoughts - discretionary
- whipped cream
- frozen yogurt
- caramel sauce

Directions:
1. Preheat stove to 400°F. Put aside a medium preparing sheet. On a medium preparing sheet, orchestrate 6 tortillas in a blossom petal design with a few creeps outside the dish and a few crawls of cover.
2. Spot a seventh tortilla in the center. Spot an enormous skillet on medium-high warmth. Include spread, slashed apples, 1/2 cup sugar and 2 tsp cinnamon. Sauté the apples for 8-10 minutes until they begin to relax, mixing normally with a wooden spoon.
3. Spoon apple blend from skillet over tortillas on prepared sheet. Spread out to make an even layer. Overlay the folds of tortilla outside the dish over the apples. Spot the eighth tortilla in the center to cover the hole.
4. Blend staying 1/4 cup sugar with 1 tsp cinnamon. Sprinkle equally over the tortillas. Spot another preparing dish on top to hold the tortillas set up and heat for 20 minutes. Expel from the stove and permit to cool for 5-10 minutes.
5. Present with discretionary frozen yogurt, whipped cream and caramel sauce. Appreciate!

Nutrition: 250 Calories 2g Fats 4g Carbohydrates

Heaven on Earth Cake

Preparation Time: 24 minutes
Cooking Time: 0
Serving: 1

Ingredients:
- 1 box Angel nourishment cake
- 1 bundle (3.4 ounces) moment vanilla pudding
- 1/2 cups milk
- 1 cup harsh cream
- 1 can (21 ounces) cherry pie filling
- 1 tub (8 ounces) Cool Whip
- 1 tablespoon almond bits, toasted

Directions:
1. Heat fluffy cake as indicated by bundle's bearings. Permit to cool and cut into 3D shapes. In a bowl, consolidate pudding blend, milk, and acrid cream and beat until smooth.
2. Put in a safe spot. In a 9x13 preparing dish, organize 1/2 of cake solid shapes layer. Spoon 2/3 of cherry over cake. Spot the staying 1/2 of the cake over pie filling.

3. Spoon pudding over cake and spread equally. Spoon and spread whipped besting over the pudding layer. Embellishment cake with the rest of the pie filling and toasted almonds. Chill for around 4 to 5 hours.

Nutrition: 250 Calories 1g Fats 5g Carbohydrates

Strawberry Upside-Down Cake

Preparation Time: 14 minutes
Cooking Time: 43 minutes
Serving: 1

Ingredients:
- 2 c. new strawberries squashed
- 2 3 Oz strawberry Jell-O
- 3 c. little marshmallows
- 18.25 oz. strawberry cake blend + fixings to get ready cake blend
- Cool Whip

Directions:
1. Take your two cups of strawberries and pound them with a fork. Fill a lubed 9x13 in cake container. Sprinkle strawberry Jell-O over the highest point of the strawberries. At that point, sprinkle the marshmallows over the Jell-O.
2. Plan cake blend, as indicated by bundle headings. Pour over the marshmallows. Heat at 350 degrees for 40-50 minutes or until cake tests are done.
3. Let sit for around 15 minutes and afterward, run a blade around the outside of the cake. Flip onto a serving plate. Refrigerate. Present with Cool Whip. Store scraps in the fridge.

Nutrition: 250 Calories 2g Fiber 1g Fats

Lemon Blueberry Poke Cake

Preparation Time: 31 minutes
Cooking Time: 63 minutes
Serving: 1

Ingredients:
- 1 box vanilla cake blend, in addition to fixings called for on box
- 2 1/2 c. Blueberries
- Juice of 1/2 lemon
- 1 tbsp. Granulated sugar
- 1/2 c. Whipped besting

For the frosting and topping:
- 1 c. (2 sticks) spread, relaxed
- 2 (8-oz.) Squares cream cheddar, mellowed
- 2 1/4 c. Powdered sugar
- Get-up-and-go of 1 lemon
- Juice of 1/2 lemon
- 1 tsp. Unadulterated vanilla concentrate
- Blueberries, for decorate

Directions:
1. Preheat stove to 350°. Line a 9"- x-13" dish with material paper and oil with cooking shower. Prepare cake as indicated by bundle guidelines. Let cool totally.
2. Make the blueberry sauce: In a little pan over medium warmth, join blueberries, lemon squeeze, and sugar. Bring to a stew and cook for 7 minutes. Expel from warm and fill a medium bowl.
3. Let cool for 15 minutes, at that point overlay in whipped beating. Make icing: In a huge bowl utilizing a hand blender, beat the spread and cream cheddar. Include powdered sugar, lemon get-up-and-go and squeeze, and vanilla and beat until smooth and soft.
4. Utilizing the rear of a wooden spoon, jab openings all over cooled cake at that point pour blueberry blend on top. Spread icing on top at that point embellish cake with more blueberries.

Nutrition: 235 Calories 2g Fats 5g Carbohydrates

Easy No-Churn Funfetti Ice Cream Cake

Preparation Time: 23 minutes
Cooking Time: 11 minutes
Serving: 6

Ingredients:
- 2 cups heavy whipping cream, well chilled
- Two teaspoons vanilla extract
- ¼ teaspoon salt
- 14 Oz sweetened condensed milk
- 2 Tablespoons unsalted butter, melted and cooled
- 1/2 cup rainbow sprinkles

For the frosting:
- 1 cup semi-sweet chocolate chips
- 1 cup butter

Directions:

1. Place a large bowl or whisk attachment into the freezer to chill for about 10 minutes. Carefully pour condensed milk and melted butter into the bowl, then gently fold into the whipped cream.
2. Then quickly fold in the sprinkles. Spread the ice cream in the prepared pan and freeze for several hours, or until firm.

Nutrition: 260 Calories 5g Fats 9g Carbohydrates

Lemon Tofu Cheesecake

Preparation Time: 44 minutes
Cooking Time: 0
Servings: 8

Ingredients:
- Silk tofu, drained – 24 ounces
- Almond butter – 1.5 tablespoons
- Date sugar – 1 cup
- Lemon zest – 1 teaspoon
- Sea salt .5 teaspoon
- Vanilla extract - .5 teaspoon
- Lemon juice - 2 tablespoons
- Cornstarch – 1.5 tablespoons
- Crust, 8-inch – 1 (optional)

Directions:
1. Preheat the oven to Fahrenheit three-hundred and fifty degrees. If you are preparing the lemon tofu cheesecake without a crust, I recommend preparing eight individual ramekins to divide the filling between. Otherwise, prepare an eight-inch crust of your choice.
2. Whisk together the lemon juice with the cornstarch to form a slurry.
3. In a food processor or blender, combine the cornstarch slurry and remaining ingredients until fully combined, smooth, and creamy. You don't want any lumps.
4. Pour the lemon tofu cheesecake filling into the prepared crust or ramekins. If baking with the crust, allow the cheesecake to cook until set, about thirty minutes.
5. Allow the cheesecake to cool to room temperature, and then transfer it to the fridge until completely chilled through.

Nutrition: 174 Calorie 2g Fat 7g Carbohydrates

Blueberry Walnut Crisp

Preparation Time: 43 minutes
Cooking Time: 38 minutes
Servings: 6

Ingredients:
- Walnuts, chopped - .25 cup
- Rolled oats - .5 cup
- Date sugar – 2 tablespoons
- Cinnamon, ground - .5 teaspoon
- Sea salt - .25 teaspoon
- Butter, cut into cubes – 2 tablespoons
- Blueberries – 4 cups
- Cornstarch – 1 tablespoon
- Date sugar – 2 tablespoons
- Lemon zest - .5 teaspoon
- Vanilla extract – 1 teaspoon

Directions:
1. Begin by preheating your oven to Fahrenheit three-hundred and fifty degrees and preparing six individual ramekins with non-stick cooking spray. Set the ramekins on a baking sheet to avoid spilling.
2. In a bowl, toss together the blueberries with the cornstarch, date sugar, lemon zest, and vanilla. Once combined, divide the blueberries between the ramekins.
3. To make the crispy topping combine the remaining ingredients with a fork or pastry cutter. It will be crumbly. Top the blueberries in the ramekins with the crumble.
4. Set the baking sheet of ramekins in the oven and bake until golden-brown, about twenty-five to thirty minutes. Remove the blueberry walnut crisp from the oven and allow the crisps to cool slightly before serving.

Nutrition: 211 Calories 2g Fats 5g Carbohydrates

Red Wine Poached Pears

Preparation Time: 37 minutes
Cooking Time: 0
Servings: 6

Ingredients:
- Bosc pears – 6
- Cherries, pitted - .5 cup (optional)
- Red wine – 2 cups
- Orange juice - .5 cup
- Vanilla extract – 2 teaspoons
- Date sugar - .5 cup
- Cinnamon stick – 1

- Cloves, whole – 8
- Orange zest - .5 teaspoon

Directions:
1. Add all of your red wine poached pear ingredients, except for the Bosc pears, into a large Dutch oven. You need a pot large enough to fit all six whole hears.
2. Allow the wine mixture to reach a simmer in the pot while stirring to dissolve the date sugar.
3. Wait until the poaching liquid has reached a simmer and then peel the pears. Place the pears into the poaching liquid, arranging them so that they are submerged.
4. Allow the pears to continue simmering on medium-low for about twenty to twenty-five minutes. But while the pears poach rearrange and rotate them every five minutes.
5. Once the pears are done poaching, keep the pears upright in the wine mixture. Remove the pot from the heat of the stove, and allow both the pears and poaching liquid to cool down together.
6. While you can serve the poached pears once cooled to room temperature
7. When chilling the pears in the fridge, keep them stored in the liquid.
8. Once you are ready to serve the pears, remove them from the liquid and set them on serving dishes. Meanwhile, add the poaching liquid into a saucepan and allow it to simmer to heat until it forms a slightly thickened syrup.
9. Pour the red wine syrup over the cold pears and serve.

Nutrition: 266 Calories 6g Carbohydrates 4g Fat

Dark Chocolate Walnut No-Bake Cookies

Preparation Time: 24 minutes
Cooking Time: 0 minutes
Servings: 24

Ingredients:
- Walnuts, chopped - .25 cups
- Coconut oil – 3 tablespoons
- Cocoa powder - .25 cup
- Dark chocolate chips - .5 cup
- Shredded coconut, unsweetened – 2 cups
- Almond butter - .5 cup
- Honey - .33 cup
- Vanilla extract – 1 teaspoon
- Sea salt - .25 teaspoon

Directions:
1. Prepare an aluminum baking sheet by covering it with kitchen parchment, wax coated paper, or a silicone mat.
2. Melt the coconut oil with the almond butter and honey over low heat in a saucepan. Once melted, stir in the remaining ingredients.
3. Use a tablespoon to scoop out portions of the chocolate walnut dough and roll each portion into a ball in your hands. Place the dark chocolate walnut no-bake cookie balls on the prepared baking sheet.
4. Freeze the cookies for ten minutes to set up. Enjoy immediately, or store the leftovers in a container in the freezer.

Nutrition: 139 Calories 14g Carbohydrates 4g Fats

No-Bake Triple Berry Mini Tarts

Preparation time: 12 minutes
Cooking time: 46 minutes
Serving: 4

Ingredients:
- Frozen mixed berries, defrosted – 1 cup
- Honey - .5 cup
- Cacao butter, melted – 5 tablespoons
- Coconut cream - .33 cup
- Walnuts, raw – 2 cups
- Dates – 1 cup

Directions:
1. In a food processor, combine the walnuts with the dates until it forms a crumbly mixture that can hold together when you press it. Scrape down the sides as needed.
2. Prepare a mini muffin tin for the crust to make the mini-tarts. Spray the pan with non-stick cooking spray.
3. Press the prepared crust into the mini muffin tin, forming mini tarts with crust pressed both on the bottom and on the sides of the muffin cups.
4. In a blender, mix the berries and other remaining ingredients until completely smooth. Divide the berry mixture between the crusts.

5. Place the filled muffin tin in the fridge and allow it to chill for six hours, or until set.
6. Use a kitchen knife to run around the edges of each tart to release them from the pan. Use a fork and take each tart out of the pan. Serve or store in a container in the fridge or freezer.

Nutrition: 239 Calories 7g Protein 27g Fats

Mocha Buckwheat Pudding

Preparation Time: 14 minutes
Cooking time: 33 minutes
Serving: 4

Ingredients:
- Buckwheat groats - .5 cup
- Cocoa powder – 3 tablespoon s
- Chocolate soy protein powder – 2 scoops
- Instant espresso powder – 1 teaspoon
- Almond butter – 2 tablespoons
- Soymilk, unsweetened - .5 cup
- Banana – 1
- Dates, pitted – 2

Directions:
1. Cover the buckwheat groats in water and allow them to soak overnight to soften. Rinse it well.
2. Add the prepared buckwheat and the remaining ingredients all into a blender together, and blend on high speed until completely smooth.
3. Serve the pudding immediately or allow it to chill first.

Nutrition: 110 Calories 3g Protein 1g Fats

Loaded Chocolate Fudge

Preparation Time: 13 minutes
Cooking time: 42 minutes
Serving: 4

Ingredients:
- 1 cup Medjool dates, chopped
- 2 tablespoons coconut oil, melted
- 1/2 cup peanut butter
- ¼ cup of unsweetened cocoa powder
- ½ cup walnuts
- 1 teaspoon vanilla

Directions:
1. Soak the dates in warm water for 20 – 30 minutes
2. Lightly grease an 8" square baking pan with coconut oil.
3. Add dates, peanut butter, cocoa powder and vanilla to a food processor and blend until smooth.
4. Fold in walnuts.
5. Pack into the greased baking pan and put in your freezer for 1 hour
6. Cut into 16 or more bite-sized squares and store in semi-airtight container in the refrigerator.

Nutrition: 120 Calories 4g Protein 3g Fats

CONCLUSION

Thanks for making it to the end of sirtfood diet cookbook. Sirtfood diet plan is a great plan that like all plans need to be implemented with a great deal of effort, discipline and determination. Sirtfood diet can help you lose weight if you fully implement it into your life and make it a habit.

As stated above this diet is not supposed to be a short-term plan but a long-term lifestyle goal. You cannot implement this diet and then revert to your normal eating habits. You need to adopt lifestyle changes. If you wish to lose weight and stay fit, then you need to do something about it.

It is suggested to eat sirtfood diet recipes every day. The future benefits of sirtfood diet will overcome any initial discomfort you might feel during the beginning phases of the diet. If you wish to make this diet successful, then you need to believe in it.

I hope you have enjoyed reading Sirtfood Diet Plan.

Good luck on your sirtfood journey!

Printed in Great Britain
by Amazon